Living w

A Resource Guide

Kathryn M. Rogers, BSN, RN, CGRN

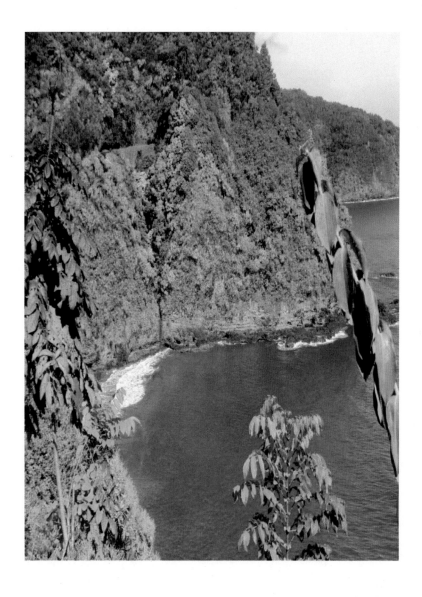

Living with Gastroparesis:

A Resource Guide

Kathryn M. Rogers, BSN, RN, CGRN

Living with Gastroparesis: A Resource Guide

Copyright 2017

All rights reserved

Title ID: 7724986

ISBN-13: 978-1981392643

To my Mom and Dad,

For always being there for me through some extremely tough times….

You never gave up HOPE, and you were my inspiration to keep on fighting!

Thank you for being the best parents any girl could ask for!

Love you Lots!!!!!!

To Bogey,

For always being right by my side every step of the way!

Thank You for choosing me to be your Mom!

You gave me hope and inspiration to keep fighting!

Love you to the moon and back, Big Guy!

To anyone fighting a chronic illness,

Never Ever Give Up HOPE!

TABLE OF CONTENTS

INTRODUCTION

Do you experience severe nausea, vomiting, or abdominal pain daily? Do you feel full quickly after eating only a few bites of food? Are you losing weight or considered malnourished? If you answered yes to any of these questions, it is highly probable that you are suffering from a delayed motility condition called gastroparesis.

Gastroparesis is a serious medical condition in which the stomach does not empty properly due to delayed gastric contractions and decreased motility issues. The stomach does not empty fast enough, resulting in serious symptoms such as extreme nausea, vomiting, abdominal pain, bloating, fatigue, weight loss, and malnutrition. There are many things that can be done to help control the symptoms. And, there is a chance that you could eventually go into remission. However, there is currently no cure for gastroparesis.

Many of us take for granted that whatever we put into our mouths will go through proper digestion without any problems. Unfortunately, there are millions of people around the world who are not able to digest foods properly. If this is left untreated, it can result in very significant issues, that could cause a downward spiral in one's health.

In this book, I will explain the condition of gastroparesis. Things that are discussed include: signs and symptoms of gastroparesis, how gastroparesis is diagnosed, different tests and procedures to expect, medications that can be prescribed, surgical options, the gastroparesis diet, coping and support groups, and listings of other resources available. In addition, I will explain this information not only from the perspective as a registered nurse who has worked in the GI lab for over thirteen years, but also as a gastroparesis patient myself.

At the age of 23, I had a rather large abdominal surgery for a very rare condition called Median Arcuate Ligament Syndrome. Basically, a ligament band was wrapped around the main arteries supplying blood to my stomach and small bowel. This presented a major problem because every time I exhaled or ate food, the blood supply to my stomach and small bowel was being cut off. If left untreated, I could have ended up with a dead gut. A vascular surgeon performed surgery to remove this fibrous band, to prevent my stomach and intestines from becoming necrotic. It was this surgery, however, that resulted in a complication called gastroparesis. I couldn't eat, lost an awful of weight, and ended up with such a severe case of gastroparesis that required a feeding tube to be placed in my small bowel for 24-hour tube feedings. I struggled with this disease for almost 10 years. I tried every medication possible for this disease, as well as, underwent multiple tests, procedures, and surgeries. Fortunately, at a time when I was the sickest, my physicians were forced to make a very risky decision regarding my health. It was this decision and risky surgery that ultimately cured my gastroparesis!

As a gastroparesis patient myself, I know exactly what you are going through. Gastroparesis is a very difficult disease that takes everything out of you. Constant nausea and vomiting can become unbearable at times, and make it extremely difficult to even get out of bed some days. Since I have dealt with this disease myself, in addition to educating many of my patients about gastroparesis during my nursing career in gastroenterology, it is my wish that this book will help you learn everything you need to know about gastroparesis. In addition, I will provide you with the knowledge that is necessary to help control the nagging, extremely bothersome symptoms associated with gastroparesis, in order to live a productive life! Remission Is Possible! Anything is possible, if you .... Never Ever Give Up… HOPE!

1

WHAT IS GASTROPARESIS?

Gastroparesis is an extremely serious medical condition in which there is significantly delayed emptying of the stomach contents. The stomach cannot empty the food into the small intestine in a timely manner. This is usually due to some sort of damage to the vagus nerve. The vagus nerve controls the movement of all food contents through the digestive tract. When there is damage to this nerve, the muscles of the stomach and intestines are prevented from functioning properly. This causes the movement of food to be delayed or even stopped/paralyzed (1).

This condition often results in chronic nausea, vomiting, bloating, fullness, early satiety, and abdominal pain. Oftentimes, patients require some form of feeding tube to ensure adequate nutrition.

Nearly 2 million Americans have been diagnosed with gastroparesis. Over 100,000 of these individuals suffer from a severe form of this disease. It is more common in women than men. And, approximately 30,000 people have a severe form of gastroparesis, called refractory gastroparesis, meaning that they do not respond to standard medical therapy. Gastroparesis can be managed medically, but there's currently no cure for this debilitating disease. It can have such a significant impact on a person's quality of life (1).

During the process of normal digestion, the stomach must contract to empty the stomach completely of food and liquids. Normally, the stomach contracts at least three times a minute. These contractions are necessary to move food through the stomach and into the small intestines within 90-120 minutes after eating. If contractions are sluggish or not as frequent, the stomach emptying is delayed. This is what results in the bothersome symptoms of nausea, vomiting, abdominal pain, bloating, weight loss, and feeling full after only eating a few bites of food.

Gastroparesis may be caused by motor dysfunction, paralysis of the stomach muscles, or it may be associated with other systemic diseases. It is most often a complication of type 1 diabetes. At least 20 percent of people with type 1 diabetes develop gastroparesis. It also occurs in people with type 2 diabetes, although less often (1).

Some additional known causes of gastroparesis include:
- Uncontrolled diabetes
- Gastric surgery causing injury to the vagus nerve
- Medications (e.g. Narcotics, Antidepressants, Opioids)
- Use of medication that blocks certain nerve signals (i.e. anticholinergic medications)
- Nervous system diseases (i.e. Multiple Sclerosis, Parkinson's)
- Amyloidosis (deposits of protein in tissues and organs)
- Scleroderma (connective tissue disorder that affects the blood vessels, skin, skeletal muscles, and organs)
- Idiopathic—meaning there is truly no known cause

Gastroparesis can be managed medically, but the disease itself has no known cure. Chronic, delayed gastric emptying can cause multiple complications including: bacterial overgrowth, bezoars, and uncontrolled blood sugar levels.

When food stays in the stomach too long, it can ferment, which eventually leads to an overgrowth of bacteria. Bacterial overgrowth is usually treated with medications.

When the food just sits in the stomach, it can harden into a solid collection/mass, which is called a bezoar. A bezoar can cause an obstruction in the stomach, which eventually prevents food from passing into the small intestine. This can be visualized during a procedure called an EGD.

A thin, flexible tube with a camera on the end is passed through the mouth down into the stomach. The gastroenterologist can attempt to remove pieces of the bezoar. However, most of the time, it is unable to be completely removed by this procedure alone. Gastroenterologists usually place the patient on some medications to help break up the bezoar. If the medications are not able to break up the bezoar, then the patient would most likely require surgery to remove it. Otherwise, the bezoar will only continue to grow and eventually block the opening of the stomach, which would require immediate surgery.

Blood sugar levels can be all over the place when food sits in the stomach. This is because blood sugar levels normally rise when food leaves the stomach and enters the small intestine. However, when the food is unable to pass into the small intestine, the blood sugar levels drop dramatically. This can make it extremely difficult for someone with diabetes to maintain adequate blood sugar levels. Even people without diabetes can feel light-headed, sweaty, and dizzy initially because the food is just sitting in your stomach and not moving forward into the small intestine. Delayed stomach emptying can make it very difficult to maintain normal blood sugar levels all the time.

One saying I always tell my patients to remember is…. "Cold and clammy…need some candy. Hot and dry…sugar high." This saying helps me to always remember what a person's blood sugar is doing just by the way they are feeling and how they appear, before even checking their blood sugar.

Normal blood sugar levels are 70-120mg/dl. When someone is hypoglycemic (low blood sugar--usually below 70mg/dl), they will appear pale and feel cold, clammy, jittery, dizzy, and even light-headed. These people need a good 4oz. of orange juice immediately to correct these symptoms. Because liquids pass much easier from the stomach into the small intestine, 4oz. of orange juice will bring their blood sugars into a normal range again quickly.

However, when someone is hyperglycemic (extremely high blood sugar), they will feel warm to the touch, appear flush, have dry mouth and skin, and most likely will be nauseated and vomiting. Decreased level of consciousness will occur when they are approaching a blood sugar level of a diabetic coma (blood sugars>400mg/dl). These individuals have way too much sugar in their blood, and they need to inject their insulin dose immediately. If they have already taken their insulin and are still having extremely high blood sugar levels, then they need to go to the nearest emergency room, or call 911. High blood sugar levels are just as deadly as low blood sugar levels. People can go into comas when their blood sugar levels are extremely high, and go unconscious when the blood sugars are extremely low.

The reason I am explaining this to you is, regardless if you are diabetic or not, with gastroparesis, blood sugar levels vary greatly because of how delayed food is when going from the stomach into the small intestines. The nutrients aren't absorbed until they are broken down by the stomach and reach the small intestine. This means that your blood sugars will bounce from being very low to extremely high and vice versa.

Remember the saying that I just taught you, "Cold and clammy… need some candy. Hot and dry…. sugar high." This should help you remember which way your blood sugar is headed, if you aren't able to check your blood sugar level with an accucheck. The easiest way to cure the symptoms associated with a low blood sugar is by drinking 4oz. of orange juice. This will raise your blood sugar levels back to within normal range quickly, and all the unwanted symptoms should go away.

Once again, if you are experiencing extremely high
blood sugar levels that do not respond to insulin, then you will need to
go to the nearest emergency room or call 911 to have this addressed.

It is much more common, though, for people with gastroparesis
(and no diabetic history) to be much more symptomatic due to low blood
sugars, rather than high blood sugars. This is because food is SO delayed
in the stomach, and your body is starving for food until it reaches your
small intestine.

Unfortunately, gastroparesis can be a very difficult
disease to live with for multiple reasons. However, there are things
medically that can be done to help your situation, which I will explain in
detail. Diet modification is one of the biggest changes that will help
control the symptoms of gastroparesis. It is possible to go into remission,
although there is currently still no known cure for gastroparesis.

2

Anatomy of the Stomach

To help you understand gastroparesis, it is important to go over the anatomy of the stomach. Your stomach is a hollow, muscular organ that processes food. It is very unique because it uses several processes to move the food along. The stomach utilizes chemical, nervous system, and electrical signals in combination to help churn, knead, and mix food with digestive juices. This results in very synchronized waves of propulsions (2).

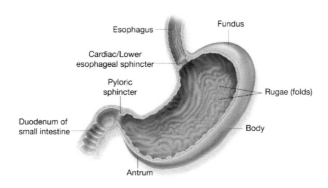

www.google.com/stomach images

Every part of the stomach has a specific function. The upper section is referred to as the fundus. It acts as the area to initially "catch" your meal. This top area gently relaxes and expands to help accommodate the amount of food you are eating.

The lower part of the stomach, called the antrum, is the vital portion of your stomach, where it converts the food into much smaller pieces. The antrum is essentially the "work-horse" portion of the stomach. As this part of the stomach churns the food into smaller pieces and eventually into a fine slurry, the antrum moves the food particles closer to the end of the stomach and through the pylorus valve. Once the food particles move past the pylorus valve, it passes into the small intestine, which is where nutrients are ultimately absorbed.

The stomach has a pacemaker region, which is situated near the body of the stomach. Lots of specialized cells in this area send out weak electrical impulses, which help to promote rhythmic, muscular action. This "pacemaker region" acts as the coordination area of the stomach. The variety of these muscular activities by the digestive systems is called "motility."

"Generally, chronic nausea and vomiting can arise from 3 sources: from the central nervous system, that is, the brain's vestibular area (middle ear); from the autonomic nervous system; or from the abdominal region (the stomach, pancreas, gallbladder/liver, or small intestine." (3)

Any problems in the function or structure in any of these areas of the stomach, can result in numerous issues, specifically chronic nausea and vomiting. Gastroparesis occurs when this system is disrupted in a way such that no contractions of the stomach or very delayed contractions occur. This results in food sitting in the stomach for hours due to the stomach's inability to grind and pump the food out into the small intestine.

Once again, gastroparesis has many different things that can cause it. Overall, the groups that make up gastroparesis sufferers are: idiopathic (36%), diabetics (29%), post-gastric surgery (13%), Parkinson's disease (7%), Pseudo-obstruction (6%), and Collagen diseases (4%). Regardless of the cause, the symptoms of gastroparesis remain the same. (3)

3

How is Gastroparesis Diagnosed?

When there is delayed stomach emptying, a person can become very symptomatic and ill-feeling. Some of the signs and symptoms associated with gastroparesis are:

- Nausea
- Vomiting
- Feeling of fullness
- Burping often
- Abdominal bloating
- Abdominal discomfort
- Acute acid reflux/indigestion
- Poor appetite
- Weight loss
- Feeling of fullness after only eating a few bites of food
- Chronic indigestion(heartburn)

Gastric Emptying Study:

The "gold standard" for diagnosing gastroparesis is with a Gastric Emptying Study. The Gastric Emptying Study evaluates how fast a pre-determined amount of food moves through your stomach and gastrointestinal (GI) tract. You will eat food that contains a radioisotope, a slightly radioactive substance, that will show up on the scan machine. The dose of radiation from the radioisotope is very small and not dangerous.

Usually the "meal" that they have you eat is either ~8oz. of watered down oatmeal, or two eggs and a piece of toast. Both meals contain the slightly radioactive isotope that allows the meal to be traced over the next few hours. After you are finished eating within the specified period, they will have you lie on your back under a machine that detects the radioisotope. An image will appear on the screen showing the food in the stomach and how quickly it leaves the stomach. Gastroparesis is diagnosed if more than half of the food remains in your stomach after 2 hours.

At times, the gastric emptying study can be combined with other studies, such as a liquid barium x-ray, barium beefsteak meal, or gastric manometry. Depending on how many tests your gastroenterologist decides on, you can expect your testing to last anywhere between 2-6 hours.

Liquid Barium X-ray:

Another way to diagnosis gastroparesis is through a Liquid Barium X-ray. After having nothing to eat or drink for 12 hours, they will have you drink a thick liquid(barium), which will coat the inside of your stomach. This will show up on the x-ray. If the x-ray shows food in your stomach, then gastroparesis is likely the diagnosis.

A normal scan would show an empty stomach after 12 hours of fasting. If the x-ray shows an empty stomach, but the doctor still suspects that you have delayed emptying of your stomach, then you may need to repeat the test on another day. A person with gastroparesis can still digest a meal normally on any given day, which could give a false test result. (4)

Barium Beefsteak Meal:

A Barium Beefsteak Meal is another possible way to detect gastroparesis. They will have you eat a meal that contains barium. This will allow the radiologist to watch your stomach as it digests the meal. The doctor gets a good idea of how well your stomach is working by watching how fast the solid food meal leaves the stomach. This test can help detect emptying problems that may not have shown up on the liquid barium x-ray. In fact, people who have diabetes-related gastroparesis often digest fluid normally, so the barium beefsteak meal can be more useful, especially in this case (4).

Gastric Manometry:

Gastric Manometry testing is the most invasive of all the testing, and is probably the most uncomfortable. This test measures electrical and muscular activity in the stomach to check for gastroparesis.

The doctor will give you some medicine through an IV to help relax and slightly sedate you for this procedure. They must be careful with how much sedation they give though, because too much narcotics will skew the results. When they feel you are at the right sedation level, the doctor will pass a thin flexible tube down your throat and into your stomach. The tube contains a wire that will be used to take measurements of the stomach's electrical and muscular activity.

When you wake up, the nurses will have you eat a small meal with this tiny wire still in place. This wire will be hooked up to a machine that will translate measurements as your stomach digests the liquids and solid food that you just ate. The measurements show how the stomach is working and whether there is any delay in digestion. The doctor will use these results to determine if there is a significant delay in the emptying of your stomach, and then come up with a plan of care.

To rule out any other causes of gastroparesis, the doctor may decide he/she would like to do an ultrasound or an upper endoscopy to check for any abnormalities that would help explain the signs/symptoms you are having.

Ultrasound:

To rule out gallbladder disease or pancreatitis as a source of the problem, you may also have an ultrasound test. This is a very simple procedure, usually performed by an ultrasound tech. He/She will use a machine that uses harmless sound waves to outline and define the shape of the gallbladder and pancreas. These images will be sent to radiology, and will be read by a radiologist. The reports will be faxed to your physician to review. The main things this test is looking for are stones in your gallbladder or bile ducts, and any narrowing or strictures in your pancreas or bile ducts. These could explain some of the symptoms too.

Upper Endoscopy(EGD):

An Upper Endoscopy (aka EGD) is an invasive procedure utilizing an endoscope to look at your esophagus, stomach, and small intestine. Although this is invasive, it is a very definitive procedure that can tell you a lot about what may be going on with your GI tract.

In pre-op, the nurses obtain a history and physical. They will explain the procedure to you as well. You will be required to tell them your allergies and all medications you take. It is most helpful if you could write down your medications on a piece of paper and bring this with you to your appointment. The nurses will need to know the name of the medication, the dose, how many times you take it, and the time of your last dose. Note: Most facilities also require a urine for pregnancy testing. Then, they will start an IV with some fluids to keep you hydrated.

After signing a consent form, you will be given a sedative through your IV. The doctor will have you lay on your left side. As you are going to sleep, the nurses will have you bite down on a bite block. It is just a thin piece of plastic that helps to protect your teeth, and the scope, during the procedure.

After you are asleep, the gastroenterologist will pass a long, thin, flexible tube (endoscope) through your mouth, and then will gently guide it down the esophagus into the stomach. Through the scope, the doctor can look at the linings of the throat, esophagus, stomach, and the beginning part of the small bowel. The doctor will be able to see if there are any strictures, ulcers, tumors, diverticulum, gastritis, etc.to help explain your symptoms. They are looking for anything abnormal, including if there is any residual food in your stomach. This will help the doctor determine which way to plan your care.

Afterwards, you will be wheeled into recovery for at least 30 minutes, where the nurses will monitor you for any side effects. After you meet the time requirements at the facility and your vital signs are stable, the nurses will remove your IV and go over discharge instructions with you and your ride. You will feel a little drowsy and loopy because of the sedation. It is required that you have a responsible adult driver with you, because you will NOT be allowed to drive home after the procedure. Most facilities will state that you are not allowed to drive, operate any machinery, no cooking on the stove, no use of power tools, no alcohol, no work, and no important legal decision making for 24 hours. This is a good time to ask for a work excuse, if needed.

Prior to discharge, the doctor will go over what he/she found. It is important that you have your adult driver with you during this time, as you probably will not remember what the doctor tells you due to the amnesic properties of the drugs given during your procedure. If biopsies (small tissue samples) were taken during the procedure, these samples get sent to a lab for analysis. The results will be back within a week or so. The doctor will go over these results with you at a follow-up appointment.

As you have read, there are many tests and procedures that can be done to check your GI tract. Specifically, for gastroparesis, the gold standard test is the gastric emptying study. While these other tests are helpful, they are not required to diagnose gastroparesis. However, it is important to rule out any other potential causes of delayed stomach emptying to make sure nothing else is going on. Once everything else has been ruled out and the "gold standard" test has been completed, your GI physician should have enough information to explain to you if you do or do not have gastroparesis. Finally, a plan should be in place as to how to proceed with your care.

4

Medications Used to Treat Gastroparesis

Once you have been diagnosed with gastroparesis, there are multiple medications that can be tried to help control your symptoms. The main types of medications you can expect to be prescribed are anti-emetics(anti-nausea), pro-motility, and anti-anxiety. Your doctor may try different drugs, or a combination of multiple drugs, to figure out what is the most effective treatment for you.

Several drugs that are used to treat gastroparesis are:

- **Metoclopramide (Reglan)-**This drug is a pro-kinetic medication used to stimulate lots of stomach muscle contractions to help empty the food faster from the stomach. It also helps reduce nausea and vomiting. Metoclopramide is usually taken 20 to 30 minutes before meals and at bedtime. Side effects of this drug are fatigue, sleepiness, anxiety, agitation, depression, and sometimes problems with physical movement. Reglan can cause some nervous system issues too because it does cross the blood-brain barrier. As a result, you may feel very jittery, anxious, or shaky. Jerk-like actions with your muscles may occur. A condition called Tardive Dyskinesia is a catastrophic side effect that can occur with prolonged use. This condition is disabling and can occur without any warning. Therefore, it is imperative that you discuss this medication in detail with your physician if he/she would like you to try this medication to treat your gastroparesis. (5)

- **Erythromycin**- Although this is an antibiotic, it is also extremely effective at improving stomach emptying times. It is a potent stimulant of solid and liquid stomach emptying. (5). This medication is best absorbed as a suspension or IV. It works by significantly increasing the stomach muscular contractions to help move food through the stomach. Some side effects of this medication are: skin rashes, abdominal cramps, light sensitivity, and abdominal pain.

- **Zithromax(Azithromycin)**- This antibiotic works a lot like Erythromycin. Either IV or suspension forms are the best. It can be taken in the AM and PM, or just once a day. Although it is an antibiotic, it causes strong stomach muscle contractions. Therefore, it helps with food digestion and motility issues. Some side effects are diarrhea, nausea, light sensitivity, and cramping. Also, prolonged QT intervals can occur with long-term use. Therefore, your physician should also monitor your heart function while you are on this medication. Note: I found this medication to be extremely helpful for myself. I was able to take this for many years without any side effects.

- **Domperidone-** This pro-motility drug is approved in Canada and other countries, but has yet to be FDA approved here in the United States. However, it is a great pro-motility drug that acts like Reglan. Domperidone is a very strong pro-motility drug that is very helpful at controlling the symptoms associated with gastroparesis. However, it doesn't have all of the nervous system side effects because Domperidone does NOT cross the blood-brain barrier. Your physician can write a script for this med, and you can get it over seas, or you can take it to a compounding pharmacy here in the US, and get it filled there. This medication usually works great, and is the one I found to work the best for many, many years. It also helps with nausea. Like Reglan, this med is taken ~30 minutes before every meal and at bedtime. The dose for an adult can be increased up to 30mg before every meal and at bedtime. Usually, they will start you out at 10mg before meals and at bedtime, and work up from there. Some side effects of this medication include: menstrual irregularities, breast engorgement, and cardiac arrhythmias. (5)

- **Phenergan-** This is a great anti-nausea medication. The doctor can write for it every 6-8 hours, or just as needed. It is available in oral, IV, and suppository forms. Phenergan really helps with nausea and vomiting. Side effects of this drug include: sedation, drowsiness, blurred vision, dry mouth. However, this is one drug that I found to truly help calm down the nausea and vomiting. Since it can make you drowsy, use with caution. Do not drive while taking this medication!

- **Zofran(Ondansetron)**-This is also a wonderful anti-nausea medication. It is one of the most powerful drugs used to help control nausea and vomiting. Zofran is not nearly as sedating as Phenergan. People who are on chemotherapy, are often prescribed Zofran. It is also available in oral, IV, SL (dissolve under the tongue) forms. The nice thing about Zofran is that you can still function when you take this, and it really does help with nausea. It can get into your system quick, if you have the form that dissolves under your tongue. It may cause some blurred vision, though, at times. Therefore, use with caution.

- **Marinol**-This cannabinoid drug comes with some controversy. It is the legal pill form of marijuana. However, GI doctors prescribe it to help with the symptoms of loss of appetite, severe nausea, and weight loss. It not only helps with nausea symptoms, but also stimulates your appetite too! Side effects are like those of marijuana: blurred vision, hallucinations, feeling high, extreme hunger, etc. Use with extreme caution. Note: You will fail a drug test with this medication on board. Therefore, make sure you have a physician's note stating that you are on this medication, if it is ever questioned.

- **Ativan**-This is an anti-anxiety medication. It is very sedating. However, it helps with the nausea and vomiting. Sometimes, GI docs will utilize this drug to help stop cyclic vomiting when nothing else works. It is available via pill or IV. Use with caution. It will cause sedation, drowsiness, blurred vision, delayed thinking, etc. Ativan can be extremely helpful in refractory cases of gastroparesis.

- **Miralax**- This is an over the counter powder medication, that is used for constipation. Most patients with gastroparesis have delayed motility overall, which can result in constipation issues. It is extremely beneficial to use a laxative, in addition to the other anti-nausea and pro-kinetic medications listed above, to help control symptoms associated with gastroparesis. This medication is typically used once a day to keep bowel habits normal and prevent any obstructions. Normal dose is 17g once a day for an adult. You can mix the powder in 8oz. of water or juice. Stir it thoroughly prior to drinking. Side effects are usually minimal. Some people may experience stomach cramping or diarrhea. Everyone is different, so be sure to discuss all your medications with your physician prior to use.

- **GERD Medications**- Prevacid, Protonix, Nexium, Zantac, Zegarid, Aciphex, etc. are all medications used to help treat and prevent gastrointestinal esophageal reflux disease (GERD). Acid reflux is very common with gastroparesis patients, because food sits in the stomach for long periods of time. Gastric acids combine with the food, and can cause severe indigestion. Delayed emptying of food results in increased inflammation along the stomach lining and esophageal lining. This can be felt as a burning sensation in your throat or stomach. Therefore, use of a medication to help prevent acid reflux, is also one of the common medications you can expect to be part of your "GI Cocktail."

- **Other Medications**--Other medications may be used to treat symptoms related to gastroparesis. For example, if you have a bezoar, the doctor may use an endoscope to inject medication that will dissolve it. And, if you have a narrowing of your pylorus (your stomach outlet to the small intestine), the MD can inject Botox into that muscle to paralyze it and keep it wide open. This allows liquids and food to move more easily from the stomach into the small intestines.

Healthcare is an evolving science. Studies are being conducted every day to discover other treatment options for gastroparesis patients. New medications and treatments will become available in the future, and I truly believe that a cure will be found for gastroparesis!

When you choose HOPE......Anything IS Possible!!!!!!

5

THE GP DIET!!

Diet modification is one of the most important things you can do when you are diagnosed with gastroparesis. This lifestyle modification is necessary. Your gastroenterologist will recommend that you eat smaller, more frequent meals, that consist of low-fat and low-fiber foods. I highly suggest that you ask your gastroenterologist for a referral to a dietician, to help you learn which foods are good to eat, and which ones you should avoid.

High fat content meals, as well as high fiber meals, are extremely difficult for a normal stomach to digest, let alone someone with delayed stomach emptying. Liquids are the easiest form of food for someone with gastroparesis to digest. Sometimes, it is necessary to go on an all liquid diet for a few days when your gastroparesis is at its worst.

The general principles for treating gastroparesis include:
- Correcting fluid and nutritional deficiencies that are occurring from chronic nausea, vomiting, and/or not being able to eat normally.
- Treating the awful symptoms that accompany gastroparesis by: dietary modifications, medications to enhance gastric emptying, and medications to reduce nausea and vomiting.
- Treat the underlying cause of gastroparesis, if possible (i.e. diabetes, thyroid disease, etc.)
- Referral to dietician to help with lifestyle and nutritional modifications.

Dietary Guidelines for Gastroparesis Patients:

♦ **Eat smaller, more frequent meals**: Eating smaller meals will decrease the distention of the stomach. In return, you may not feel as full or bloated, and your stomach should empty quicker. However, to maintain adequate nutritional intake, people with gastroparesis need to eat 4-6 smaller meals per day. It is recommended that once gastroparesis is diagnosed, a dietician appointment is made to help discuss and explore your tolerance of solids, semi-solids, and liquids, as well as dietary balance, meal sizes, and timing of meals. (6).

♦ **Avoid foods with a high fat content:** Fatty foods take longer to empty from the stomach. By consuming less fat-containing foods, the stomach won't take as long to empty. However, some fat-containing liquids, like Boost and milkshakes, may be tolerated since they are liquids. These fat-containing liquids are ok to help provide the necessary calories and nutrition needed. (6).

♦ **Eat low fiber foods:** Fiber, overall, delays gastric emptying and can cause constipation. While it is good for a normal person to eat a lot of fiber, this is the opposite with gastroparesis patients. The fiber may end up binding together and cause a blockage or a bezoar. Some high fiber foods to avoid include: oranges, green beans, potato peels, apples, berries, broccoli, corn, nuts, and seeds. (6).

♦ **Drink fluids at the end of the meal. Avoid carbonated beverages:** Gastroparesis patients have a limited amount of space in their stomach for food. To get the best nutrition possible, save the liquids for last. Make sure you eat the foods that will give you protein and calories first. Then, proceed to the liquids at the end. The only time this doesn't work is if a patient is on an all liquid diet. If this is the case, obviously, liquids can be had at any time. However, do not drink any carbonated beverages as this will cause stomach distention, and irritate your gastroparesis even further. (6)

♦ **Do not lie down for 1-2 hours after eating:** To prevent terrible acid reflux and further delayed stomach emptying, make sure that you are awake and upright up to 2 hours after eating. Try to take a walk within 1-2 hours after eating to help aide in the digestion process. (6).

♦ **Take a multivitamin once a day:** Try to get in the habit of taking one multivitamin once a day, to help with nutritional deficiencies. Multivitamins do come in liquid forms, which would be the best for gastroparesis patients. Other nutritional supplements may be necessary, but should be monitored closely by your treating physician. (6).

If despite these recommendations, you are still having continued delayed gastric emptying symptoms to the point that you are vomiting multiple times a day, then your physician may decide to either admit you to the hospital for fluid resuscitation, or place you on an all liquid diet for a few days until this period of gastroparesis subsides.

It is unique that stomach emptying of liquids is usually normal in patients with gastroparesis. A liquid diet can very often not feel very satisfying, though. However, there are some very interesting combinations you can come up with when you put your mind to it. Skim milk, carnation instant breakfast, milkshakes made with skim milk and low-fat frozen yogurt, yogurt, low-fat puddings, low-fat ice cream, custard, smoothies, juice drinks, crystal light, etc. are all options that fall into the liquid category. To meet the nutritional needs and caloric intake requirements that your body needs, sometimes prepared drinks like Boost, Ensure, or even baby foods need to be considered. Oftentimes, these supplements will give you a lot of calories and protein, with little volume.

Despite these attempts at dietary interventions and medications, patients with chronic symptoms of gastroparesis may still end up with severe dehydration and malnutrition. Occasionally, these refractory patients need an alternative method to obtain adequate nutrition and fluids to survive. This might involve delivering fluids and nutrients directly into the small intestine using a jejunostomy tube (J-tube), which bypasses the stomach.

A J-tube is semi-permanent. It is placed surgically, and must remain in place for a minimum of 6 months. The physician orders tube feeds to run through this tube.… either all the time, every couple of hours, or as a bolus feed several times a day. These tubes can be removed if nutrition improves significantly, and the patient is able to eat enough nutrients by mouth again.

A nasojejunostomy tube (NJ tube) is like a j-tube, however, it is placed down the nose and resides in the small bowel. This tube is only temporary, though. However, it is a good tube to try if the physician is thinking about placing a more permanent tube, such as the j-tube. The NJ can "buy" the patient time, to help give them the nutritional support they may need if their gastroparesis is exacerbated due to say a viral illness. It can remain in place for ~2 weeks. This may be just the right amount of time to get a person back on track, without having to place the more permanent j-tube. I will discuss these tubes more in depth in the surgical section.

In the most severe cases of gastroparesis, where the stomach and entire intestines are basically paralyzed, the only choice available for nutritional support at that point is through intravenous fluids and 24-hour TPN (total parenteral nutrition). These patients do not tolerate anything by mouth, because their stomach and intestines are non-functional due to being paralyzed. TPN is basically a bag full of all the nutrition, electrolytes, and calories a person needs in a day.
While it is difficult to live off TPN, it is possible. The physicians can change the formulas of the TPN to include more lipids, more fat content, more electrolytes, etc. to tailor to the needs of the patient.

Gastroparesis patients need a dietician to help them learn about what they can and cannot eat. They can help you plan small meals throughout the day. Oftentimes, it takes some creativity to eat well, without becoming bored with the same foods. It is often trial and error too…. what may work for one person, may not work for another. Below is a basic guide for gastroparesis patients, as far as what foods they can eat and what foods should be avoided. (7).

GASTROPARESIS DIET GUIDELINES:

Food Group	Foods to Eat	Foods to Avoid
Milk Products	Skim milk, low fat or fat free yogurt, pudding, or cheeses	2% milk, whole milk, sour cream, heavy whipping cream, half and half, regular cheese
Soups	Soups made from skim milk or fat free broth	Soups made with cream, whole milk, or broths containing fat
Fruits	Canned fruits without skin, fruit juices, applesauce, peaches, and pears	All raw and dried fruits, canned fruits with skins (apricots, cherries, plums, blueberries, fruit cocktail, oranges, grapefruit, pineapple, persimmons)
Meats	Egg whites, creamy low-fat peanut butter, poultry with skins removed, lean fish, lean beef	Bacon, sausage, bologna, salami, hot dogs, goose, duck, canned beef, spare ribs, organ meats, fish packed in oil, regular peanut butter, steaks, roasts, chops, dried beans, lentils
Fats/Oils	Consume in moderation butter, margarine, and cooking oil	Regular salad dressings, nuts, olives, avocados, coconut, lard
Breads/Grains	White breads, low	Oatmeal, whole

	fiber cereals, cream of wheat, pasta, white rice, egg noodles, low fat crackers	grain starches, egg bagels, Chinese noodles, croissants, donuts
Vegetables	Tomato juice, well cooked vegetables without skins (acorn squash, beets, carrots, mushrooms, potatoes, spinach, summer squash, strained tomato sauce, yams)	All raw vegetables, cooked vegetables with skins (broccoli, brussel sprouts, cabbage, cauliflower, celery, corn, eggplant, onions, peas, peppers, pea pods, sauerkraut, turnips, water chestnuts, zucchini, beans (wax, green, lima)
Condiments	Fat free gravy, mustard, ketchup, BBQ sauce	Gravies, meat sauces, mayonnaise
Desserts/Sweets	Angel food cake, low fat puddings, fat free frozen yogurt, Jell-O	Cakes, pies, cookies, pastries, ice cream, fruit preserves
Beverages	Gatorade, diet soft drinks, coffee, tea, water	Milk shakes, alcoholic beverages

A Sample Meal Plan for Gastroparesis Patients:

Breakfast: 1 cup cream of wheat cereal
½ cup skim milk
½ cup grape juice
1 scrambled egg
Snack: 10 ounces of instant breakfast with skim milk
Lunch: ½ cup vegetable soup
½ turkey sandwich
½ cup applesauce
½ cup skim milk
1 tablespoon miracle whip
Snack: 10 oz. banana shake (made with 1 banana, 1 small
plain or vanilla yogurt, 8oz. skim milk)
Dinner: 2-3 ounces baked chicken or fish
½ cup mashed potatoes
1 teaspoon margarine
½ cup spinach
½ cup skim milk
½ cup canned peaches
Snack: ½ cup fat-free pudding, custard, or Jell-O

6

GP TREATMENTS/PROCEDURES

Once gastroparesis is established as a diagnosis, your GI physician may need to intervene with a more invasive procedure, at times, to help control your symptoms of nausea, vomiting, and abdominal pain. I already talked about an Upper Endoscopy (aka EGD) earlier, as a procedure that may need to be done. Another procedure that you might need to have done is an EGD with pyloric dilatation, or an EGD with Botox injection into the pylorus. Both procedures are done exactly like a regular EGD. However, it is during the EGD where the different techniques take place.

EGD with Pyloric Dilatation or Botox:

An EGD w/pyloric dilatation or Botox is an invasive procedure utilizing an endoscope to look at your esophagus, stomach, and small intestine. During the procedure, the doctor will use a pyloric balloon placed through the endoscope to stretch open the pylorus, which will ultimately help the food and fluids drain easier into the small bowel. OR, he/she may inject Botox into the pylorus muscle to paralyze that muscle and keep it open for food and fluids to drain easier into the small bowel. It is up to the doctor which intervention he/she will do. And, it can also be dictated by the insurance company as well, unfortunately. This is what happened to me.

I initially had EGD's w/Botox for several years until insurance started denying it because "Botox is not FDA approved for gastroparesis." So, my MD had to change to doing EGD's w/pyloric balloon dilatation. Both procedures worked very well for me. I will admit though, the times my pylorus was injected with Botox lasted much longer than the stretching with the balloon. I typically would get complete relief of symptoms for ~12 weeks with the Botox, and usually ~8-12 weeks with the pyloric balloon dilatation.

To help prepare you for these procedures, here is a scenario as to what to expect for an EGD w/Interventions:

In pre-op, the nurses will have you change into a gown, and will ask you to have a seat on a cart. They will obtain a history and physical. You will sign a consent form for the procedure and anesthesia. Then you will be required to tell the nurses your allergies, and list all the medications that you take. It is most helpful if you could write down your medications on a piece of paper. The nurses will need to know the name of the medication, the dose, how many times you take it, and the time of your last dose. In addition, please write down any conditions you have been diagnosed with and what surgeries you have had done in the past. An IV will be started with some maintenance fluids. <u>Note:</u> Most facilities also require a urine for pregnancy testing currently too.

When it is your procedure time, the techs/nurses will wheel you into a procedure room, and hook you up to a monitor. They will monitor your vital signs the entire time. You will most likely be placed on some oxygen. When people are sedated, they do not breathe as deep. So, this is a precaution that most facilities do as a standard.

The doctor will have you lay on your left side. They will place a bite block in your mouth (it is just a piece of plastic that you bite down on….it protects your teeth and protects the scopes too). You will be given a sedative through your IV. Most facilities are now trending towards Propofol, a medication that is quick acting and wears off faster vs. Fentanyl and Versed (conscious sedation). After you are given a deep twilight sleep, he/she will pass a long, thin, flexible scope in your mouth, and then will gently guide it down your esophagus, stomach, and the first part of your small bowel.

Through the endoscope, the doctor can look at the linings of your GI tract. The doctor will be able to see if there are any strictures, ulcers, tumors, diverticulum, gastritis, etc. in your esophagus, stomach, or first portion of your small bowel. Then, the doctor will either use a pyloric balloon through the scope to stretch the pylorus, or inject Botox into the pylorus muscle to paralyze that muscle, which will cause it to remain wide open. The MD may also take some biopsies (tissue samples) to send to the lab to check for an infection or any tissue abnormality. This usually just takes a few minutes total. I would say that 99.5% of my patients never remembered anything about the procedure, and were comfortable during the scope.

After the procedure is finished, you will be wheeled into recovery for at least 30 minutes, where the nurses will monitor your vital signs and observe you for any side effects from the procedure. After you meet the discharge requirements at the facility and your vital signs are stable, the nurses will go over discharge instructions with you and your ride. You will feel a little drowsy and loopy because of the sedation. It is required that you have a responsible, adult driver with you, because you will NOT be allowed to drive home after the procedure. The doctor will go over what he/she found. And, then you will be discharged home with follow-up instructions. Because of the sedation, most facilities will state that you are: not able to drive, operate any machinery, no cooking on the stove, no use of power tools, no alcohol, no work, and no important legal decision making for 24 hours. Just go home, watch some tv, and rest up. The medications will wear off over the next 24 hours.

If you experience any problems such as chest pain, severe abdominal pain, or fainting, please call 911 and go to the nearest emergency room. Complications from these procedures are rare, however, they do occur on occasion. It is extremely important to get immediate help if any of the above symptoms occur after your procedure.

7

Total Parenteral Nutrition(TPN)

Sometimes, gastroparesis symptoms can become so severe, that your doctor will need to admit you to the hospital. It isn't uncommon to have "gastroparesis flares" due to a viral illness, or any other illness. When your body is fighting another illness, such as the common cold, this can set you back and increase your gastroparesis symptoms significantly. Nausea and vomiting may become so severe, that your physician may decide he/she feels you need to be admitted to the hospital for fluid resuscitation and IV nutrition.

If this episode lasts only temporary, receiving IV fluids and "gut rest" may be all that your body needs at that time. However, viral illnesses are known to exacerbate symptoms of gastroparesis, which can set you back several weeks with an inability to eat or drink enough fluids. When this happens, your physician may decide to offer nutrition through a central line (a thin catheter that is placed into a large chest vein).

Total Parenteral Nutrition(TPN) allows the doctor to deliver nutrients directly into the bloodstream, and completely bypasses the digestive system. A bag of nutrition called TPN, will be run through your central line. The nutritional fluid appears white, and it enters your bloodstream through a large central vein. Typically, a dietician, pharmacist, and doctor will decide on what exactly needs to be placed in your bag of nutrition each day. TPN usually includes all of the necessary electrolytes, proteins, lipids, fats, and anything additional your body is lacking at the time. TPN is usually run over either 12 hours or 24 hours. This allows for complete "gut rest." (8).

Total Parenteral Nutrition(TPN):

TPN is normally given through a large central vein. A catheter is inserted into the chest area under local anesthesia and sterile conditions. Oftentimes, the placement of a central line is performed in an operating room. This helps to decrease the chance of infection.

Several different types of catheters are used. The determining factor as to which catheter is used, is the expected duration of use.
The catheters are made of silicone. Once the catheter is in place, your doctor will order a chest x-ray, to make sure the placement is correct.
TPN is typically administered in a hospital. However, under certain

circumstances, and with proper education, it may also be used at home for long-term therapy.

TPN solution is mixed daily by pharmacists under extremely sterile conditions. Maintaining sterility is essential for preventing infection. For this reason, the outside tubing leading from the bag of solution to the catheter is required to be changed daily, and special sterile dressings that are covering the central line catheter are also required to be changed every other day under sterile conditions.

"The contents of the TPN solution are determined based on the age, weight, height, and the medical condition of the individual. All solutions contain sugar (dextrose) for energy and protein (amino acids). Fats (lipids) may also be added to the solution. Electrolytes such as potassium, sodium, calcium, magnesium, chloride, and phosphate are also included, as these are essential to the normal functioning of the body. Trace elements such as zinc, copper, manganese, and chromium are also needed. Vitamins can be included in the TPN solution, and insulin, a hormone that helps the body use sugar, may need to be added. The TPN catheter is used only for nutrients; medications are not added to the solution. Adults need approximately 2 liters of TPN solution daily, although this amount varies with the age, size, and health of the individual. Special solutions have been developed for individuals with reduced liver and kidney function. The solution is infused slowly at first to prevent fluid imbalances, then the rate is gradually increased. The infusion process takes several hours." (8).

TPN therapy requires daily monitoring of a patient's weight, as well as frequent checks of: blood sugar levels, labs, electrolytes, blood gasses, fluid intake, urine output, and monitoring of waste products in the blood (i.e. plasma urea). TPN is very hard on a person's liver and kidneys. Therefore, daily monitoring of liver function and kidney function tests also need to be obtained in the daily labs. The contents of the TPN solution are then individualized every day based on the results of these tests. (9).

While a patient has a central line in place, patients, as well as caregivers, must be alert to any signs of infection, including: fever, redness, swelling, abnormal drainage, and increased pain at the catheter site. The biggest complications that can occur with central line placement includes: infection, pneumothorax (air in the lung cavity), and blood clots. Ideally, TPN will provide all the nutrients in the correct quantity needed, to allow the body to function properly. However, risks can occur because of the TPN too. These risks associated with TPN use include:

- Metabolic imbalances—i.e. hypoglycemia (low blood sugar levels)-Occurs when TPN is stopped abruptly.
- Fluid imbalances—can lead to major organ failure
- Infection

Other References:

Al-Jurf, Adel S. and Karen Dillon "Indications for Total Parenteral Nutrition (TPN)." *University of Iowa Virtual Hospital.* March 2003 [cited 16 February 2005]. ⟨http://www.vh.org/adult/provider/surgery/totalparenteralnutrition⟩.

"Drug Information: Total Parenteral Nutrition." *Medline Plus Medical Encyclopedia.* 1 April 2003 [cited 16 February 2005]. http://www.nlm.nih.gov/medlineplus/druginfo/medmaster/a601166.html.

"Nutritional Support: Total Parenteral Nutrition." *The Merck Manual.* Eds. Mark H. Beers and Robert Berkow. 1995–2005 [cited 27 February 2005]. http://www.merck.com/mrkshared/mmanual/section1/chapter1/1c.jsp

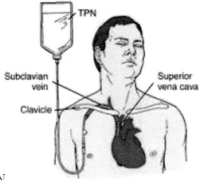

*www.google.com/*TPN

Total Parenteral Nutrition is usually only used as a temporary method to help get you through a difficult spell of gastroparesis. There is a very high risk for infection while being on TPN. Sterile technique is always to be used while accessing your central line. The healthcare providers will monitor your vital signs and labs closely to make sure you are not developing an infection from this form of nutritional feeding.

While TPN is usually only temporary, some people with gastroparesis may have such a severe case of it, that this is the only form of nutrition available to them. This is an extremely rare case of gastroparesis; however, I know people who have no choice but to live off TPN because their digestive tract does not function properly at all.

Although extremely rare, it is possible for a patient's entire stomach, small bowel, and large bowel to become completely "paralyzed." This means that the body is not able to tolerate any food or fluids by mouth at all! Patients who have this type of severe, refractory gastroparesis, the only option available for their nutrition and hydration is total parenteral nutrition.

Lots of education on TPN and central line care can be performed prior to discharge, as well as at home. This allows these types of refractory gastroparesis patients to live as much of a normal life as possible at home. Prior to discharge, a case manager will be assigned to your situation. They will come and talk to you about where you live, what your medical/physical needs will be, and if you need assistance with normal every day activities at home. Case managers will work with your insurance company, and arrange for all of the necessary equipment and supplies needed to be delivered to your home prior to discharge. This way there is no lapse in your care.

Medical equipment will be arranged to be set-up at your home, and nurses can be scheduled to come out and help with your IV line and TPN care. While it may be inconvenient to be hooked up to IV fluids and IV nutrition all the time, this therapy could very well save you from being admitted frequently to the hospital due to dehydration after a severe bout of gastroparesis. It is possible to live a normal life at home, if you must receive total parenteral nutrition.

8

Enteral Therapy:

NJ, J-tubes, and Venting G-tubes

Sometimes it is necessary to explore other options when medications, dietary modifications, and fluid resuscitation or parenteral nutrition fail to control your symptoms of gastroparesis. Many physicians feel that placing you on TPN long-term has too many risks. However, your body needs the nutrition and electrolytes to survive. If you are unable to keep anything that you eat down, or have severe, persistent nausea and vomiting despite all medical therapy, your MD may suggest a temporary way to provide nutrition through a feeding tube called a nasojejunal tube (NJ tube).

An NJ tube, is a thin, flexible tube that is passed through your nose and guided down into your small bowel. The doctor will first numb your nose with a numbing gel. Then, he/she will slowly feed the thin tube down your nose and guide it all the way down through your stomach and then into your small intestine using x-ray guidance or fluoroscopy. Once the NJ tube reaches the portion of the small bowel, called the jejunum, this is where the tube will be fixed in place for tube feedings to work properly.

The doctor will inject a very tiny amount of dye through the NJ tube to verify the correct placement, and then they will place a small holding device on your nose, as well as tape to your cheek, to ensure that the tube stays in place. The placement of the NJ is a little painful and irritating. Some doctors may give you a little sedation to help relax you as they attempt to place the NJ tube properly.

Since an NJ tube bypasses the stomach and resides in the small intestine, tube feedings will be able to be started without causing you any nausea or vomiting. A dietician will help decide which tube feeding formula will be the best formula for your body's needs. The doctor will decide to either run the tube feedings only a few times a day as "bolus" feeds, or run them as continuous feeds all the time (24-hour feeds), or only run them in the evening (nocturnal feeds). It all depends on how dehydrated and malnourished you are at the time, as well as how much rest the doctor feels that your stomach needs.

An NJ tube is usually very temporary….no more than a few weeks. It can become very irritating to your nose, and the back of your throat. I've had an NJ multiple times, and within a few days, the back of my throat would become so ulcerated and sore from the tube resting on the mucosa. It became very difficult to swallow at times.

The nurses will follow your doctor's orders, and will administer the tube feedings as prescribed. The bottle of tube feedings is hung on an IV pole and attached by tubing through a feeding pump. The tail end of the tubing attaches to the NJ tube just outside of your nose. The nurse will also "flush" your NJ tube periodically to prevent the tube from clogging. This is a very necessary step, because if the tube clogs, then it may have to be replaced all over again. There is a thing called "clog buster" that the doctor can try first before removing the clogged tube. However, if they are unable to get it unclogged, the doctor will have to remove the tube and either place another NJ tube, or discuss other options.

Most of the time, an NJ tube can "buy" you enough time to help you over the hurdle when you are having a severe gastroparesis flare. After 1-2 weeks, the NJ tube will be removed, and the doctor will either allow you to try and begin eating again, or he/she will discuss a more permanent solution for your gastroparesis symptoms and malnutrition, such as a jejunostomy tube (J-tube).

www.google.com/NJtubefeedings

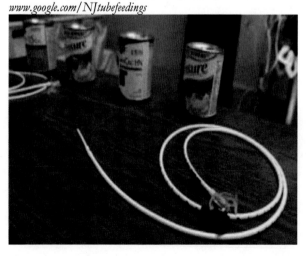

How the NJ is secured in place

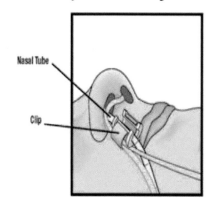

Nasal Tube

Clip

www.google.com/NJtubefeedings

Jejunostomy Feeding tube(J-tube)

If other approaches that we've discussed do not work, and the doctor feels you will require additional nutritional support over time, he/she will most likely refer you to a surgeon for placement of a Jejunostomy tube(J-tube). A j-tube is inserted under general anesthesia. While you are asleep, the surgeon will place the j-tube through the skin on your abdomen into the small intestinal area called the jejunum. This feeding tube allows for nutrients and hydration to go directly into the small intestine, bypassing the stomach altogether. Since you are bypassing the problem area (the stomach), gastroparesis patients usually do very well tolerating j-tube feedings.

You will receive special liquid supplements to use with the j-tube. A dietician will work with you and your physician to determine which formula will be the best option under your circumstances. Usually, the tube feeds are started at a low rate, and increased every day very slowly. This allows the small intestine time to adapt to the tube feeds, without overwhelming your system.

Initially, you may feel some bloating and gas. This is normal, as your body hasn't been receiving nutrition daily and must remember how to work properly again. Therefore, the tube feeds are gradually increased.

A jejunostomy tube is extremely helpful when gastroparesis prevents the nutrients and medications from reaching the bloodstream. By avoiding the source of the problem (the stomach), and putting nutrients and medications directly into the small intestine, these products are digested properly and delivered into your bloodstream very quickly. A jejunostomy tube can be temporary or more permanent, depending on your gastroparesis symptoms. Because abdominal surgery is involved, a j-tube is reserved for patients with severe, refractory gastroparesis.

Jejunostomy Tube:

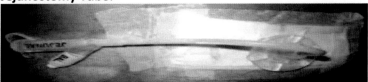

www.google.com/jejunostomy/tube

What happens after the procedure?

After the procedure, an antibiotic ointment is usually applied on the tube site, and a dressing is placed over the j-tube. Once your vital signs are stable and you meet discharge criteria from the PACU, your nurse will give report to the floor nurse. Then, you will be taken to your hospital room. The nurses will take good care of you, and monitor your surgery site, as well as, your vital signs. You will be placed on some pain medication after surgery to help control your pain levels.

Once you are awake and the anesthesia has worn off, a dietician and a nurse will teach you how to use your j-tube for feeding, how to use a feeding pump, how to take care of the j-tube at home, and suggest what feeding solution is the best for you at that time. Tube feeding is started by your primary care team once you have met certain goals after surgery.

Examples of J-tubes:

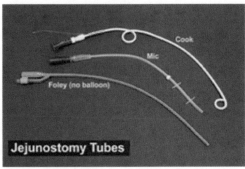

www.google.com/jtubes

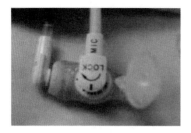

www.google.com/ low-profilej-tube

Low-profile J-Tube: Can be placed after initial j-tube tract is in place. After ~4-6 months of initial placement, MD can change to flat, low-profile mic-key tube.

Checking, Cleaning, Dressing, and Securing the J-tube:

- **Check the skin around the tube daily.**
-Look for skin redness, swelling, and note any drainage
-Alert the primary care team of any pain around your j-tube site

- **Clean the skin around the tube daily and anytime there is leakage around the tube.**
-For 4-6 weeks after a J-tube is put in, bath water should not be so deep that the tube is under water. If you take a shower, the water should fall on your back only.
-Ask your doctor when you can bathe or shower normally.
-Wash your hands before and after cleaning the j-tube site.
-If dressings are used around the tube, these must be removed and discarded first.
-Use a clean wash cloth or cotton balls to wash the skin around the tube with only a mild soap and water.
-Clean the j-tube with soap and water also during this time.
-Use cotton tip swabs to clean hard-to-reach places.
-Rinse your skin and be extremely careful and make sure you dry you skin around the tube site extremely well.

- **Dressing the J-tube:**
-For the first few days after placement, if there is any drainage, you will need to cover the area with a dressing.

--J-tube sites that are healed and not draining may be left open to air. If you continue to have small amounts of drainage though, then you need to place a split 2x2 or 4x4 gauze dressing under the tube to prevent skin irritation.

- **Securing the J- tube:**
  -A tube that is left hanging, will pull on the bowel tract. Over time, this can injure the tract and the inside of the intestines. There are several ways you can secure the jejunostomy tube:
  *Tuck the tube gently into your clothing.
  *Make a tape tab on the tube, then pin through the tape tab to the inside of your clothing.
  *Use paper tape to safely secure the tube.

- **Using the J-tube for feeding:**
  -Feedings through a J-tube are always done using a feeding pump. A visiting nurse or home healthcare company will help arrange for your feeding pump, and they will give you instructions on how to use the pump correctly at home. They will also be available to assist you in caring for your tube at home.

- **Flushing the J-tube:**
  *To reduce the risk of tubes clogging, always flush with at least ~30ml of lukewarm water:
  *Before and after each intermittent feeding
  *Before and after giving any medicine through the tube
  *Flush every four to six hours with continuous feeds
  *Whenever feeding is interrupted
  *Every day if the J-tube is not being used

- **Medicines through the J-tube:**
  -If you are giving medications through the J-tube, it is very important to flush the tube with 30ml of water between each medication, and after the last medication to ensure all the medications are passed through the tube completely.
  -You do not want the medications to mix with each other or mix with the feeding in the tube. This may cause your tube to become clogged.
  -Use a liquid form of the medicine, if possible. If you must use solid medicines, be sure to crush them finely and mix with water. If in doubt, ask your pharmacist if your

medicines can be crushed.
-Never add medicines to a tube feeding formula. Use a syringe to add the medicine directly through the feeding adapter.

Dealing with J-tube problems:

What if the J-tube falls out?
-Cover the abdominal J-tube site with a clean gauze pad. Tape in placed. Then, call your surgeon immediately to arrange for a new tube to be placed. They may send you to the ER to see if the original tract can be saved.

What if the J-tube becomes clogged?
-If the tube becomes clogged, try alternating between flushing with warm water and aspirating with the syringe. When you aspirate with a syringe, simply pull back on the plunger of the syringe while it is connected to the feeding tube. Call your home care nurse or surgeon if the tube remains clogged after 4-6 attempts over the period of an hour.
-There is a "clog buster" that can be used, but isn't always successful. Your MD may be able to unclog the tube using this medication.

What if I have connection problems with the tubing?
-If the tip of the feeding tube set does not stay securely in place with the j-tube, use a cotton tip swab moistened with water to "scrub" the inside of the feeding tube adapter. This helps to remove any oils that may have built up. Also, the tip of the feeding tube set may need to be cleaned out.
-Try to replace the feeding tube adapter, and change the tubing set.
-Call your home healthcare nurse if these steps do not help.

When do I need to call the doctor?

Problem	Action
Fever, chills, nausea, severe vomiting; Redness or swelling around the tube site; Bleeding around the tube site.	-Call your doctor immediately. -Go to the nearest emergency room, if you cannot reach your doctor. -These are all signs and symptoms of an infection. Lab work will need to be drawn, and antibiotics will most likely need to be started.
Hard abdomen or severe abdominal pain	-Call your doctor immediately… most likely, they will tell you to go to the nearest emergency room to rule out an obstruction, infection, or perforation(rupture) of the bowels. -Do not eat or drink anything in case you need emergency surgery.
The tube becomes dislodged or clogged (tube will be extremely difficult to flush)	-Call your doctor immediately. -Dislodged tubes must be replaced quickly (within 1-2 hours) or the j-tube site will close. -Your physician may instruct you to go to the emergency room. The ER can place a temporary "Foley" catheter into the tract, if the site hasn't already closed. Then, your surgeon can place another j-tube, when available. -Clogged tubes are not usually an emergency, however, they will need to be replaced as soon as possible. Your MD may try to place a clog buster down the tube to try and break up the clogged tube. If unable to do that, then the j-tube will need to be replaced. -Try to remain hydrated…drink plenty of water and Gatorade, if possible, since you are no longer getting tube feeds until the J-tube is replaced.

Lastly, if you continue to have severe nausea despite everything we have already talked about, another thing that your GI doctor may recommend is a venting gastrostomy tube(G-tube). This tube can be placed easily during an upper endoscopy procedure, with the help of a surgeon. Although this is considered rare, this tube can be placed for "venting" or "decompressing" the stomach to help alleviate nausea and vomiting symptoms. <u>The G-tube does not bypass the stomach; therefore, it should not be used for tube feedings at all.</u> The g-tube will be attached to a Foley bag, which will help collect drainage of bile and other acidic contents from the stomach. This is usually not performed as much, however, I wanted to mention it to those who may be desperate for relief as this could be used as one of the last resort items.

G-tube (also known as a PEG tube) for Venting purposes only:

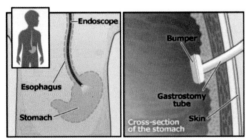

PEG Procedure

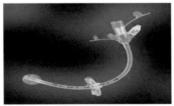

www.google.com/gtubeventing

9

Surgical Options for Gastroparesis

Surgery intervention is usually reserved for the most difficult, severe gastroparesis patients, as well as, those with refractory gastroparesis. There is currently very limited data available regarding success rates with surgical treatment of gastroparesis (10). Therefore, surgery should only be utilized as a last resort, as it is a permanent situation that could lead to other life-threatening diseases such as Dumping Syndrome.

Surgery options for patients with severe refractory gastroparesis includes: gastric electrical stimulation, surgical pyloroplasty, venting/g-tube, jejunostomy tubes, gastrectomy, surgical drainage procedures, and pancreatic transplants in diabetic patients. The most common surgical procedures for gastroparesis is gastric electrical stimulation(GES), pyloroplasy, and j-tube feeding tube placement. The other surgical procedures are performed as a very last resort after careful evaluation in patients with profound gastric paralysis (10).

Gastric Electrical Stimulation(GES)/Gastric Pacemaker:

GES allows "electrical stimulation to be delivered by two electrodes usually placed laparoscopically onto the serosa surface of the stomach overlying the pacemaker area in the body of the stomach. Leads from the electrodes connect to a pulse generator that resembles a cardiac pacemaker. The pulse generator is placed into a subcutaneous pocket of the anterior abdominal wall. The pulse generator delivers low energy pulses at a frequency of 12 cycles/minute." (11). These pulses help to generate movement of the food contents from the stomach into the small intestine. Overall, it is used to help increase gastric emptying times, as well as, control all the symptoms associated with gastroparesis.

The most common implantable gastric stimulator is called *Enterra therapy*, which is made by Medtronic Inc.

What is Enterra® Therapy?

Enterra® Therapy is a recent gastroparesis treatment that has been approved by the FDA as a device available specifically for the treatment of gastroparesis, when conventional drug therapies are not effective. The Enterra Therapy device is called a gastric electrical stimulator(GES).

This gastric electrical stimulator uses mild electrical pulses to stimulate the lower stomach (antrum) to contract. It is a fully implantable system that consists of two unipolar intramuscular leads (thin wires) and a neurostimulator. Since the neurostimulator can be turned on or off, the physician can terminate Enterra® Therapy at any time. (12). You can go to Medtronic's website to see this actual device at:

www.medtronic.com/patients/gastroparesis/device/index.htm

GES Surgery:
"A small medical device called a neurostimulator is implanted under the skin, usually in the lower abdominal region. Two insulated wires called leads are implanted in the stomach wall muscle and then connected to the neurostimulator. The procedure is performed under general anesthesia.

The neurostimulator sends mild electrical pulses through the leads to stimulate the smooth muscles of the lower stomach. This may help to control the chronic nausea and vomiting caused by gastroparesis.

After the device is implanted, the doctor uses a handheld, external programmer to adjust the neurostimulator and customize the stimulation. Stimulation can be adjusted without surgery. The stimulation can be turned off by the doctor at any time if the person experiences any intolerable side effects." (11)

Benefits of GES:

"Gastric electrical stimulation uses mild electrical pulses to stimulate the smooth muscles of the lower stomach. This may help to control the chronic nausea and vomiting associated with gastroparesis of a diabetic or idiopathic origin when drugs haven't worked.

A clinical study (WAVESS – Worldwide Anti-Vomiting Electrical Stimulation Study[1]) using the Enterra® neurostimulator for treating nausea and vomiting has shown that most, but not all, patients have some relief of their vomiting symptoms." (11)

Risks of Surgery:

Implanting a gastric electrical stimulation device carries the same risks as those associated with any other gastric surgery. The risks of GES surgery include:

- Bleeding
- Infection
- Perforation of the stomach
- Allergic response to implanted materials
- Temporary or permanent neurologic complications
- Pain at the surgery site, that may be permanent
- Bruising at the device pocket site
- Chance the device does not provide relief
- Device malfunction requiring additional surgery

Possible Side Effects of Gastric Electrical Stimulation Surgery include:

- Gastrointestinal (GI) symptoms—abdominal cramping
- Abdominal pain
- Feeding tube complications
- Difficulty swallowing or dehydration
- Acute diabetic complications
- Loss of therapeutic effect

Possible Device Complications include:

- There may be pain, infection, lack of healing where the gastric electrical stimulation parts are implanted.
- The gastric electrical stimulation parts may wear through your skin, which can cause an infection and/or scarring.
- The GES device could stop working because of mechanical and/or electrical problems. Either of these would require additional surgery.
- Your body may have an allergic reaction to the gastric electrical stimulation device. Your body could also reject the system (as a foreign body).
- The lead may perforate your stomach, or device components may become entangled with or obstruct other internal organs, requiring immediate emergency surgery.
- There is the possibility of tissue damage resulting from the stimulation settings or a malfunction of one of the parts of the gastric electrical stimulation device.

GES Surgery

What to Expect:

Gastric electrical stimulation is intended to reduce symptoms of chronic, drug-refractory nausea and vomiting associated with gastroparesis of idiopathic or diabetic origin. However, gastric electrical stimulation is not a cure. Although not all patients will benefit from gastric electrical stimulation, for those that do, the rate of improvement will vary from person to person. Due to this newly discovered therapy, the long-term effectiveness of the gastric pacemaker device is not documented at this time.

Before the Surgery:

Prior to surgery, your doctor will have you undergo some pre-op testing, which usually includes: blood work, EKG (to look at your heart function), and undergo a history and physical. During this time, the pre-op team will ask you about any medical history, prior surgeries, how well you tolerate anesthesia, any allergies, any medications you take, etc. It is very helpful if you can list your allergies, medications (include dose and frequency/day), medical history, and surgical history on a piece of paper, and keep this with you always.

Your doctor will discuss the entire surgical plan with you, and answer any questions that you have. Implanting a gastric electrical stimulation system usually takes ~1-2 hours, and is performed under general anesthesia. This means you will be completely asleep during the surgery, and should not feel anything. Your surgeon will determine the best locations for the incisions, as well as, the placement of the GES device and leads. These locations are based upon your unique anatomy, medical history, and what your personal preference may be.

During the Surgery:

Your surgeon will attempt to place the device in an area that is most comfortable for you, and allow you to maintain your normal daily activities. In addition, he/she will follow special implant and programming considerations if you have another medical device already implanted (like a pacemaker or spinal cord stimulator).

You can anticipate that the surgery will last ~1-2 hours. Based on your surgeon's preference, one of two surgical approaches will be used for your device implant:

- Laparotomy or "open approach" – surgery is performed through a small abdominal incision
- Laparoscopy – special surgical instruments are inserted through small incisions to perform the procedure

During the surgery, the electrode at the tip of each lead is placed in the muscular wall of your stomach. The lead bodies are then routed under your skin, from your stomach to the gastric electrical stimulation device. These leads will then be connected to the GES device.

The small device (looks like a pacemaker) is placed into a pocket that the surgeon will create just beneath your skin. It is usually placed below the rib cage and above the belt line in the lower abdominal region. The device pocket is then sutured closed. Once the surgery is completed, you will then be taken to the PACU, where nurses will keep a close eye on you as you begin to wake up from the anesthesia.

As you begin to wake up, you will most likely be sore and possibly nauseated from the surgery. The nurses will obtain orders from the doctor for pain medications, as well as, anti-nausea medications, if needed, to keep you comfortable. They will monitor you for at least an hour or longer, until you meet the criteria to be discharged. It is up to your physician if you stay overnight, or if he/she feels you are stable enough to go home that day.

As stated before, implanting a gastric electrical stimulation device has risks related to the surgical procedure itself, including infection, discomfort, or bruising at the pocket site. As well as, risks related to the therapy and device itself.

After the Surgery:

After the surgery, your doctor will ask the clinical programmer to adjust your GES device settings to a level that is appropriate for your needs. Programming is non-invasive and can be done in the hospital or doctor's office at any time via a "remote."

It is normal to have some pain at the site for ~2 to 6 weeks after the surgery. Be sure to follow the instructions that you are given at discharge. You will need a responsible adult with you, as you will not be allowed to drive home because of the anesthesia. It is recommended that you have someone at home with you, who can help you. You will be drowsy from pain medications, and sore from the surgery. Due to post-op restrictions, you will need someone to help you with normal activities of daily living.

During your post-op recovery, be sure to follow your doctor's advice. Avoid heavy lifting or any activities that involve excessive or repetitive bending, twisting, bouncing, or stretching for up to 8 weeks. These movements could damage or displace your leads. Displacing the leads would affect the GES device's ability to provide adequate stimulation to the correct areas of your stomach.

Please note, you should not feel the stimulation from your GES device. It is very important to call your doctor if previous symptoms return, or if you have new or unusual abdominal pain, cramping, nausea, or vomiting. These symptoms may indicate a problem with your implanted system, and require immediate attention. (13).

Check-ups and Monitoring:

To maintain the most effective control of your symptoms, your doctor usually can adjust the GES settings during an in-office programming session. Your doctor will schedule follow-up visits to monitor your progress. A typical follow-up schedule may include office visits at 1 week after surgery; then 1, 3, and 6 months after the surgery. If everything is ok at 6 months, then your visits would change to just as needed after that. Be sure to keep these follow-up appointments because they provide multiple opportunities for device assessment, and the GES system can be adjusted, if necessary. (12).

If you move, make sure you give your doctor your new address. Make sure to carry your device registration card with you at all times, and also make a copy of the card for each of your health care providers (doctors, dentists, physical therapists, nurse practitioners, etc.). It is imperative that you contact the device registry if your address or physician changes, as they need to know your address at all times in case of recalls or device issues.

Please discuss any questions or concerns that you have about potential risks, complications, and side effects of GES with your surgeon. It is imperative that you truly understand what the doctor intends to do, and exactly what is involved. This is an invasive surgery; however, it could change your life for the better. Always try to weigh the risks and benefits. If the benefits outweigh the risks, the GES may be a good option to give you your life back!

When to Call Your Doctor:

Be sure to contact your doctor with any questions you have regarding your GES device, medications, physical activity, diet, follow-up visits, or any other concerns. Contact your doctor if you are *not* experiencing the same symptom relief from the GES device, that you previously experienced. If you have a flare-up of gastroparesis symptoms, try not to be alarmed, as settings can be adjusted.

Contact your doctor immediately if:

- You are not receiving adequate therapy for your symptoms. Your GES device may simply need readjustment to a different setting, or there may be a problem with one of the leads or the neurostimulator.
- You experience any uncomfortable pulsating or stimulation sensations in your abdominal area.
- You have new or unusual abdominal pain, cramping, nausea, or vomiting at any time after surgery.
- You have severe pain, redness, or swelling at the incision site.
- You experience any other unusual symptoms.
- You are considering other dental or medical procedures

After gastroparesis is diagnosed, medications are usually the first line of treatment to stimulate proper stomach contractions. Diabetics will be encouraged to control their blood sugar levels, to help alleviate symptoms of nausea and vomiting. Patients with a history of using narcotic medications will be instructed to reduce their use of those drugs, as this may help alleviate the condition.

Diet modification is the biggest priority with gastroparesis. Eliminating fatty foods, eating low-fiber meals, eating smaller, more frequent meals are all things that are encouraged to help control gastroparesis symptoms. However, despite these lifestyle modifications, sometimes gastroparesis symptoms may continue to persist. Patients with persistence of symptoms despite medical intervention, are considered to have "refractory gastroparesis."

If your physician diagnoses you with severe or refractory gastroparesis, and you are not a candidate for a gastric pacemaker, your doctor may recommend a surgery called a pyloroplasty. This surgery involves surgically opening the tightened pylorus valve at the end of the stomach. This surgery makes this change permanent.

A pyloroplasty essentially does what an EGD w/Botox or EGD w/pyloric dilatation does, except it makes that opening permanent. A pyloroplasty widens the opening at the end of the stomach. In theory, by making the outlet of the stomach larger, it allows food and liquids to move easier out of the stomach and into the small intestine for absorption of necessary nutrients. Like any surgery though, there are risks. However, if benefits outweigh the risks, a surgical pyloroplasty may be a good option for you.

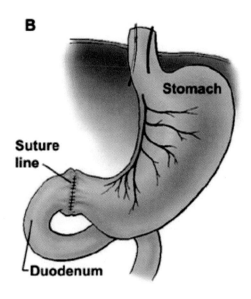

B

Stomach

Suture line

Duodenum

www.yoursurgery.com

Pyloroplasty

Pyloroplasty is a surgical procedure that is performed to widen the opening in the lower part of the stomach(pylorus), so that stomach contents can empty into the small intestine (duodenum).The pylorus is a thick, muscular area. When it thickens, food cannot pass through very easily, which causes the symptoms of nausea, vomiting, fullness feeling after only eating a few bites of food, etc. A pyloroplasty widens the opening at the end of the stomach permanently.

The surgery is done while you are under general anesthesia. You will be completely asleep for this surgery. Surgery will last approximately 1-2 hours. The surgeon will make a cut in your abdominal area. If the surgery is done using a laparoscope, three smaller cuts can be made, which makes recovery easier.

The surgeon will cut through some of the thickened pylorus muscle, so the pylorus becomes wider. The cut is then closed in a way that keeps the pylorus open. This allows the stomach to empty its contents faster. The outside abdominal incision is usually closed with either sutures, steri-strips, derma bond, or staples depending on how big the incisions are. (14).

Risks of a Pyloroplasty:

- Adverse reactions to medications
- Problems breathing
- Bleeding
- Infection
- Damage to the intestine
- Hernias
- Leakage of stomach contents
- Long-term diarrhea
- Malnutrition
- Tear in the lining of nearby organs (mucosal perforation)
- Dumping Syndrome

After the Surgery:

After surgery, the health care team will monitor your breathing, blood pressure, temperature, heart rate, pain levels, and your intake/output. The average hospital stay is usually 2 - 3 days, although if you are doing well, your doctor may discharge you earlier. While you are in the hospital, your doctor will order pain medications to keep your pain level under control and help keep you comfortable. You can expect to have a pretty sore belly, especially at the sites of your incision. And, it will take some time for you to build your abdominal muscles up again. The doctor must cut through some of your abdominal muscles to get to the stomach, therefore, these muscles must heal again. You may feel pain in your back too, and it is usually just in compensation for what all your body has been through.

After surgery, they will have you on IV pain meds or a PCA pump that will allow more autonomy in controlling your pain. Then, they will transition you over to oral pain medications prior to leaving the hospital. You will most likely be on some antibiotics too, as prevention for infection. When you wake up from surgery, you'll notice that a tube is placed down your nose (called a NG tube). An NG tube is normally hooked up to suction to help decompress your stomach. This will be in place to keep your stomach contents empty and help to control nausea until your bowels wake up. Once you have bowel sounds, and no nausea, the doctor or nurse will remove this NG tube, and start you on a clear liquid diet.

A clear liquid diet usually consists of beef broth, chicken broth, sprite, water, and apple juice. If a clear liquid diet is tolerated, then they will slowly progress you to full liquids, soft foods, and then return you to a normal gastroparesis diet.

The nurses will also be in frequently to monitor your vital signs, assess your abdomen and surgical sites, give you your medications, and monitor for any complications. Be sure to report anything that is abnormal or any issues that you are having. It is common to have constipation after surgery on the belly, therefore, the doctor will most likely order a stool softener to help keep your bowels regular.

It is imperative that you do the exercises as recommended by your physician, nurses, and physical therapists. Usually, the post-op instructions will include that you do hourly deep breathing exercises, as well as use an incentive spirometer (a device that you take deep breaths into). The incentive spirometer will help prevent you from getting pneumonia. You will be sore after the surgery, and it is normal to not take exceptionally large breaths. However, this predisposes patients to infection and pneumonia. So, it is standard for physicians to order this incentive spirometer device to use every hour while you are awake.

In addition, you may also have some sequential devices (or SCD's) on your lower legs. This is used to prevent blood clots. The nurses will also encourage you to move your ankles around in circles and push them up and down, while you are lying in bed. Sedentary activity, such as lying in bed all day, can set you up for a serious complication called a DVT (deep vein thrombosis), which is a fancy word for a blood clot in your legs.

Blood clots are very serious, and could potentially break off from your leg and travel to your lungs and/or brain, which could potentially cause a pulmonary embolism, heart attack, or stroke. So, it is extremely important that when you are lying in bed, make sure that you do your leg exercises and keep the sequential devices(SCD's) on while resting. Once you start feeling a little better, the nurses and therapists are going to want to get you up and walking. The more you can get up and walk with assistance, the faster you will heal.

It is normal to have some pain at the site for ~2 to 6 weeks after the surgery. Be sure to follow the instructions that you are given at discharge. You will need a responsible adult with you, as you will not be allowed to drive home because of the anesthesia. It is recommended that you have someone at home with you, who can help you. You will be drowsy from pain medications, and sore from the surgery. Due to post-op restrictions, you will need someone to help you with normal activities of daily living.

During your post-op recovery, be sure to follow your doctor's advice. Avoid heavy lifting or any activities that involve excessive or repetitive bending, twisting, bouncing, or stretching for up to 8 weeks. Lifting heavy objects after abdominal surgery is dangerous. You can tear your sutures open, cause damage to your bowels, and potentially tear a muscle, which is extremely painful. If your sutures or staples come apart, you need to contact your surgeon immediately, because of the risk of infection and need for immediate surgery to close the wound again.

The best thing you can do during your recovery is rest, relax, and enjoy the time you have off from your normal everyday life. It is imperative that you follow your discharge instructions, keep your follow-up appointments, and continue to do your home therapy to heal properly. Once you are completely healed, and you obtain your physician's approval, most patients can return to normal every day activities within 6-8 weeks. Returning to work depends on your occupation and what your position requires your body to do all day long. It will remain up to your doctor to determine any further restrictions as far as work goes, as well as when it is safe for you to return to work.

There is one last thing that I need to mention while recovering from any gastric surgery. Anytime you have surgery on your stomach, there is the potential for a pretty serious complication called "Dumping Syndrome."

10

Dumping Syndrome

Dumping syndrome is common after any gastric surgery, but especially after a pyloroplasty. "It is a group of symptoms that may result from having part of your stomach removed or from other surgery involving the stomach. The symptoms range from mild to severe and often subside with time. Although you may find dumping syndrome alarming at first, it is not life threatening. You can control it by making changes in what and how you eat. By controlling dumping syndrome, you will also be avoiding the foods that tend to make you gain weight." *(15)*.

After a pyloroplasty, food can move through the wider opening at the end of the stomach very quickly at times. As a result, food contents are rapidly "dumping" into the small intestine. Certain foods are known to trigger these symptoms such as: refined sugars, dairy products, fatty and fried foods. Therefore, it is recommended to stay away from these products if you experience symptoms of dumping syndrome.

Dumping syndrome may occur ~30-60 minutes after you eat. Early phase symptoms can last about an hour and may include:

- A feeling of fullness, even after eating just a small amount
- Abdominal cramping or pain
- Nausea or vomiting
- Severe diarrhea
- Sweating, flushing
- Rapid heartbeat
- Dizziness or light-headedness

Late phase dumping syndrome may occur as well. When this happens, it usually occurs ~1-3 hours after eating. Symptoms may include:

- Weakness or extreme fatigue feeling
- Flushing, sweating, or rapid heartbeat
- Shakiness, dizziness, light-headedness, or fainting spells
- Loss of concentration and/or mental confusion
- Feelings of hunger

Symptoms of late phase dumping syndrome occur because of widely fluctuating blood sugar levels. Remember, blood sugars rise once food enters the small intestine. Therefore, when you have food entering rapidly into the small intestine, as is the case with dumping syndrome, this causes a rapid rise and fall in blood sugar levels.

Follow the steps below to help reduce the symptoms of dumping syndrome *(15)*:

- Avoid eating sugars and other sweets such as: candy, soft drinks, sweet juice drinks, cakes, cookies, pastries, and sweet breads (i.e. donuts, coffee cake, etc.).
- Avoid all dairy products and alcohol.
- Avoid eating solids and drinking liquids at the same meal.
- Avoid drinking liquids 30 minutes before and 30 minutes after meals.
- Use fiber supplements, such as Metamucil, Citrucel, or Benefiber.
- Use sugar replacements, such as Splenda, Equal, or Sweet 'N Low, instead of regular sugar.
- Try to eat more complex carbohydrates (i.e. Vegetables, whole-wheat bread), instead of simple carbohydrates (i.e. Donuts, sweet rolls, and ice cream).
- Be sure to drink more than 4 cups of water and/or other sugar-free, decaffeinated, non-carbonated beverages throughout the day to prevent dehydration.

What can you eat with Dumping Syndrome?

- Eat 5-6 small meals or snacks a day.
- Eat small portions (i.e. 1 oz. of meat, or 1/4 cup of vegetables).
- Remember to cut your food into very small pieces and chew well before swallowing.
- Combine proteins or fats along with fruits or starches. (For example, combine fruit along with cottage cheese.)
- Stop eating when you first begin to feel full.
- Drink liquids 30 to 45 minutes after meals.
- Laying down after eating may help prevent dizziness/fainting

It is extremely important to manage dumping syndrome so that you stay well-nourished, and don't lose a lot of additional weight. Be sure to discuss any symptoms you have with your doctor, to see what else they can do to make your lifestyle more tolerable. Sometimes, medications or additional surgery may be necessary to help correct the severe symptoms of dumping syndrome. (15).

11
Associated Conditions:
MCAS and Celiac Disease

There are two associated conditions with Gastroparesis, that I learned from Dr. Chopra. He said that they are finding that MCAS and Celiac Disease are highly associated with Gastroparesis.

MCAS (MAST CELL ACTIVATION SYNDROME):

MCAS (Mast Cell Activation Syndrome) is an immune condition in which mast cells inappropriately and excessively release chemical mediators into the blood stream, resulting in a range of chronic symptoms including: anaphylaxis attacks, cardiovascular, dermatological, neurological, respiratory, and gastrointestinal problems.

There is no known cause, but this condition appears to be inherited. Symptoms of MCAS are caused by excessive release of chemical mediators by mast cells. These mediators include leukotrienes and histamines. This condition may be mild, until exacerbated by stressful events, or symptoms may develop and slowly trend to worsen with time. This condition can be difficult to diagnose, especially since many of the numerous symptoms may seem to be considered "vague." Many patients see specialist after specialist, before being diagnosed correctly with this condition many years later. (16).

Common symptoms include: flushing, easy bruising, either a reddish and/or pale complexion, itchiness, light-headedness, dizziness, pre-syncope, syncope, diarrhea, cramping, intestinal discomfort, nausea, vomiting, swallowing; throat tightness, "brain fog", headaches, migraines, congestion, coughing, wheezing, conjunctivitis, general fatigue, food/drug/and chemical intolerances, heat/cold intolerance, osteoporosis and/or osteopenia. (16).

Diagnosis of MCAS can be difficult. It can be diagnosed through an EGD with biopsy of the esophagus. If many mast cells are found on the biopsy, then MCAS is diagnosed. However, lack of knowledge by many medical professionals, is currently an issue for obtaining proper diagnosis. (16).

Treatment includes: Mast cell stabilizers (Cromolyn Sodium), H1-antihistamines (Zyrtec, Ketotifen) and H2-antihistamines (Zantac, Pepcid), and Antileukotrienes (Singular). (16).

Dyes, fillers, and binders in many medications are often the culprit in causing MCAS reactions. Compounding pharmacies should be considered. (16).

Lifestyle changes may also be needed as well to avoid triggers. Avoidance of triggers is extremely important. It should be emphasized that MCAS patients can potentially react to any new exposure, including foods, drinks, medications, microbes, and smoke. (16).

A low histamine diet and other elimination diets, such as Celiac disease diets, can be helpful in identifying foods that trigger or worsen symptoms. Most MCAS patients already have high histamine levels, so ingesting foods with a high histamine level can worsen symptoms such as vasodilation that causes faintness and/or palpitations. (16).

CELIAC DISEASE:

Celiac disease is also known as a gluten-sensitivity. It is an immune reaction to eating gluten, which is found in wheat, rye, barley, and oats.

If you have Celiac disease, eating gluten triggers an immune response in your small intestine. This reaction results in damage to your small intestine over time, and prevents absorption of nutrients. The intestinal damage causes fatigue, diarrhea, weight loss, bloating, and anemia.

There is currently no cure for Celiac disease, however, following a strict gluten-free diet can help manage your symptoms and promote healing in your small intestine.

Symptoms of Celiac disease can vary greatly. However, the most common signs and symptoms are diarrhea, weight loss, fatigue, bloating, gas, abdominal pain, nausea, constipation, and vomiting. Other symptoms may include: anemia, osteoporosis, itchy/blistery skin rash, mouth ulcers, headaches, fatigue, joint pain, acid reflux, lactose intolerance, and cognitive impairment. (17).

Diagnosis of Celiac disease is done by a biopsy of the small intestine during an EGD. If flattening of the villi is found in the biopsy, diagnosis of Celiac disease is made.

If you are diagnosed with Celiac disease, you will need to avoid all foods that contain gluten. Ask your doctor for a referral to a dietician, who can help you plan a healthy, gluten-free diet. You'll need to make sure to include enough vitamins, fiber, nutrients, and calcium in your diet.

People with Celiac disease must avoid: barley, bulgur, durum, farina, graham flour, malt, rye, semolina, spelt, triticale, and wheat. Packaged foods should be avoided unless they are labeled gluten-free. Cereals, pastas, and baked goods (breads, cakes, pies, and cookies) usually contain gluten and should be avoided. Other packaged foods that may contain gluten include: beer, candies, gravy, meats, seafood, processed lunch meats, soups, salad dressings, sauces, and soy sauce. (17).

Foods that you are allowed to eat include: fresh foods, fish, and poultry; fruits, most dairy products, potatoes, vegetables, wine and distilled liquors, ciders, and spirits. Certain grains and starches are allowed in a gluten-free diet including: amaranth, arrowroot, buckwheat, corn, cornmeal, gluten-free flours (rice, soy, corn, potato, and bean), pure corn tortillas, quinoa, rica, and tapioca. (17).

Fortunately, Celiac disease is becoming more and more recognized by the manufacturers. An increasing number of gluten-free products are becoming available. Udi is one of my most favorite brands of gluten-free foods.

12

A Story of HOPE!

As a child, I was an extremely active, healthy little kid. I was always extremely thin, however, I never had any major health issues at that time. I had a broken bone here and there from playing soccer, but for the most part, there was nothing major bothering me all the time. However, as a teenager, I began to have some issues with my stomach.... feeling full quickly, heartburn, and nausea here and there. I was also having near-passing out episodes, fainting spells, and I kept saying that "something just doesn't feel right." My pediatrician ran some labs and tests, and always felt that I had some "underlying" condition that he just couldn't put his finger on. After coming up with no answers for my symptoms, my pediatrician referred me to a cardiologist.

I began my cardiologist around the age of 18, just at the time I was out of high school and transitioning into college. I was accepted at Miami University in Oxford, Ohio, where I would go on to receive a BSN in Nursing.

During college, I continued to have these "episodes" where I just didn't feel right.... cool clammy hands, blurry vision, nauseated, light headedness, racing heart rate, sweating, and near passing out/fainting episodes. These symptoms came on without any warning....I would be fine one minute, and the next I'd be struggling to stand up and walk a straight line. It got so bad at one point that I always was looking at my surroundings to see where I could "land" if needed, with these episodes.

Since I was away at college, it made it difficult to diagnose any problems because my cardiologist was seeing me from a distance, and titrating changes over the phone. During my initial consultation, my cardiologist felt that I had what was called "vasovagal syncope." Basically, this meant that the part of my nervous system responsible for regulating blood pressure and heart rate was malfunctioning. My body would go into these fits where my heart rate would go high, and my blood pressure would go low as a result. That is what was causing the near-fainting episodes. We tried multiple medications, in addition to salt loading.

I was instructed to do "salt loading" where I was constantly eating salty foods and drinking a ton of water at the same time. With the extra salt on board, it theoretically helps to retain the water. The extra fluid would help my blood pressure to not drop so low. There were other things that I had to do when I had these episodes such as lay flat with my feet elevated above my heart. How cool did that look as a college freshman who kept near-passing out, and had to either put my head down below my knees while sitting on a chair, or lay flat on the ground and elevate my feet above my heart? Luckily, I was in the nursing program, so when I had these "episodes" my classmates knew what was going on, and could help me, as needed.

Despite these changes, I was continuing to have these episodes of near-fainting, and just didn't feel right. I changed cardiologists, and had multiple tests run. Finally, after nothing was showing up, my cardiologist took a drastic measure and placed a "loop recorder" in my chest. Basically, the purpose of this was to constantly be able to see what my heart was doing all the time, and pinpoint if there were any abnormal heart beats, etc. Well, within the first 24 hours of having the loop recorder placed, I had an episode. I was at home with my Mom and we were putting some dishes away. I remember that I reached over my head to put some dishes on the shelf. Well, that's all it took to set off one of these weird episodes.

I remember telling my Mom that I was having an episode, and I went into the living room to sit down. I had to put my head down on the table, because I was SO dizzy and nearly passed out. But, I remained awake during the entire episode, which lasted about 2 minutes or so. My Mom said all the color in my face was gone, and I was extremely pale, clammy, sweating, etc.

The next morning, I called my cardiologist's office and told them that I had one of my so called "episodes." They asked for me to come in right away, so they could pull the information off the loop recorder. I remember that day very clearly. The nurse was very kind, and hooked me up to a bunch of wires. She downloaded the loop recorder information. She looked at me and said, "Did you lose consciousness during this?" I told her, "No. But, I felt like I was pretty close to."

It turns out that my heart was completely stopping…. that is what was causing my "episodes." Test, after test, after test…and we finally had an answer. My cardiologist looked at the EKG, and said that my heart stopped for 8 seconds. My heart rate went from a completely normal rhythm in the 70's, then dropped drastically to the 50's, changed into another junctional rhythm in the 30s, and then stopped for 8 seconds. But, my heart restarted after that to a normal, but slow heart rhythm in the 50's. (Normal heart rates range between 60-100 beats/min.). So, this meant that I needed a pacemaker. A pacemaker at the age of 23? Seriously????

The cardiac surgeon who did my surgery was Dr. Charles Love. He is the best cardiac surgeon ever, and said that I was one of his youngest patients to ever receive a pacemaker for what they ultimately decided was "Sick Sinus Syndrome." A very rare, irregular rhythm that resulted from my heart conduction system malfunctioning.

Once the pacemaker was in place, it really resolved most of the near-fainting episodes. They did have to increase my heart rate to 90 beats/min. continuously to keep my blood pressure up due to the vasovagal syncope issues as well. However, with time, things settled, and this was the least of my issues!!!!

Imagine having to have a pacemaker placed at the age of 23. During one of the most important time periods in your life as you just graduated from college, you're getting ready to start your new career, buy a new house, and really learn how to live on your own. A time when things are supposed to settle.... get married, have children, and love life.

I had started my nursing career in the Surgical Intensive Care Unit(SICU) at The Ohio State University in Columbus, Ohio. As a new graduate, I was just getting my life started. I moved back home to Columbus, Ohio and rented an apartment on a golf course at Little Turtle Golf Club in January of 2002. That is also when my first furry friend came into my life.... named "Bogey."

Bogey was my rescue dog from the Franklin County Animal Shelter. I adopted him 1/8/2002. He was the most beautiful golden retriever ever, with the sweetest personality. Whoever his previous owners were, lost an amazing dog. I can't imagine how devastated that family must have felt, when they lost their dog for whatever reason. I am extremely grateful for how much time and effort went into training him. Bogey was completely potty-trained, never barked, and had some signs that he may have been an agility trained dog. I know that family must have been completely devastated when they lost their dog. However, I gained the most beautiful, loyal companion ever. For $35, I brought Bogey home and he was my best friend and guardian angel.

Bogey chose me that one day. When I was walking around the animal shelter with my Mom, I was looking for a specific female dog that I had seen online. We did find her...she was a young, Irish Setter. However, when she was let out of her kennel.... away she ran down the hallway and she didn't want anything to do with me. I was kind of bummed at the time, but everything happens for a reason. My Mom encouraged me to continue looking through the three different holding areas, to see if another dog would be a better fit.

As I turned the corner in the second holding area, I remember my eyes saw the most beautiful, young male golden retriever with a shaved down fur coat. He was laying just as quiet as possible in his kennel. His front paws were crossed, and his head was lying down on the cold floor.

"Look Mom…. HE's beautiful!" I said.

A huge smile overcame my face. I scanned his ID card quickly…. "Young Male Golden Retriever, approximately 1-2 years old." He had been in the shelter for 3-4 days already. I looked at my Mom, and she looked at me. We knew instantly, and we were both thinking the same thing…. this may be it! This may be the dog that I was meant to take home!

Then, his tail thumped multiple times on the ground as I bent down to get a closer look at this gorgeous dog, with the most beautiful eyes and the most gorgeous, shiny golden fur coat. This young male dog with his big, brown eyes looked up at my face. I gave him a big smile back.

"HI there! What's your name???" I asked.

His tail thumped even harder and faster on the floor. I knew I wanted to let him out, and check out his personality. Other people were circling around the kennel area at the same time. I needed to get the attention of one of the pound keepers before anyone else did first. Just as I went to stand up, this precious dog placed his right paw on the front of his kennel door….it was priceless! This was the moment that melted my heart for "Bogey."

My family always grew up with female golden retrievers, and have always found these types of dogs to be the best breed ever. This beautiful, young, male golden retriever caught my eye immediately, and stole my heart as soon as he put his right paw up on the kennel door as I was walking by. It was as if he was saying, "STOP! Please…Take me home! I will make you the happiest person ever!"

This dog was amazingly beautiful….too beautiful and too perfect to be left at the pound. How did he even get here in the first place? If only dogs could talk……

I had some reservations about male dogs and heard they could be very territorial and pee on things. I remember my Mom saying though, "Just give him a chance. Male dogs can be very loyal, especially if it is only You, as a female owner." It was at that moment I decided I wanted to meet this beautiful boy. So, I had my Mom guard this dog's kennel to prevent someone else from seeing him before I could get to an employee there to let him out of the cage.

I caught the attention of an employee fairly quick, and asked for them to come and let this beautiful golden retriever out of his kennel so that I could meet him. As soon as the kennel door opened, this sweet boy immediately wagged his tail and laid in my lap. He licked my hands and face, as if he was giving me kisses. This was it! He had me at hello! Things happen for a reason…. that day, it was meant for the two of us to meet!

Prior to leaving, I had to fill out some paperwork and the lady at the counter says to me, "What's your dog's name?" Hmmm…. I hadn't planned to name him quite yet. However, it was required for me to provide a name to this person for registration purposes.

After a little hesitation and some thought, I named him "Bogey." I don't know how or why I came up with that name. However, he had to have a name for me to take him home. So, I had very little time to consider a name for this dog. "Bogey" came to my mind though. At the time, I was getting ready to move into my apartment that was right on a golf course. However, I was not a golfer at all and I always told my family that I could kick the ball further than I could hit it! So, the word "bogey" wasn't far from my vocabulary at the time.

This was a beautiful dog that was left behind at a pound, but would go on to do so many amazing, wonderful things, and truly lived each day to its fullest. So, while his name sort of comes from the game of golf, it also is in honor of one of the best actors ever, Humphrey Bogart. Looking back on this now, even though it was a name that I had to give the animal shelter extremely quickly, "Bogey" was a perfect name for this most perfect dog!

Since I was coming home with a dog, this meant that my time was being cut short with living in "transition" with my parents. I was ready to move and start my new life as a nurse, in a new home, with a new dog. I moved into my own apartment in January of 2002. I adopted Bogey on 1/8/2002. He was my New Year's baby….my loyal, beautiful, protective, furry companion!!

Those first few weeks were rough, as Bogey adjusted to my schedule, and I adjusted to be a new nurse in an incredibly difficult intensive care unit. Lots of stress occurred over the next two years, while I learned the ropes of being a new nurse and taking care of extremely sick surgical patients daily.

My work hours were very strange. I worked 12 hr. shifts, but since I was a "newbie," that meant I was mandated to work overtime when we were short staffed. This meant my 12-hour work days would turn into an agonizing 16 hour day, sometimes. Unfortunately, much of this time, Bogey was left by himself in a large, open kennel. This wasn't fair to him, and soon I learned this wasn't the best fit for me, either. Working 16 hr. days took a toll on my body…. big time! I was working until 3:30am some days, however, by the time I gave report to the next nurse, and walked out to the parking lot and drove the 30 minutes home….It was easily going on 5am.

Poor Bogey didn't understand why I was gone so long, and his days and nights became mixed up, as well as, mine too. Initially, I had to help him deal with severe separation anxiety, which I totally expected with a dog that was just picked up from the animal shelter. Bogey also had a terrible fear of any male person, and became very submissive under these conditions, and would rollover and pee when any guy would pet him. My younger brother and Dad helped to get Bogey out of that frightful stage, and Bogey loved everyone after that…. a little too much! Bogey wouldn't hurt a fly, and he thought everyone was his friend!

Bogey had been through everything with me, and was always there through thick and thin. He is the one who kept me going when my health took a turn for the worse. I swear this dog was SO smart, and knew exactly what I was saying when I talked to him. He tried to talk back, by using his vocal cords to "talk" in his own sweet way. Our bond grew tremendously over his last 12 years. He kept me going during some extremely difficult times in my life. I am forever grateful for that extremely special, beautiful, loyal dog who "chose" me that cool winter day many years ago.

I wanted to let you know about my special bond with my amazing dog, Bogey, to let you know how important it is to have that "outlet" and someone to turn to when you need someone to just listen, unconditionally. The things I am about to tell you, will help you understand why it was SO important for me to have such a loyal companion by my side during some extremely difficult periods in my life.

As I told you a little bit ago, I had to have a pacemaker placed at the age of 23, which is just about unheard of. I can't give you the exact statistics on it. I just know that my cardiologist said I got the award for being his youngest patient ever to receive a pacemaker. Initially, it scared me knowing that my heart was truly "stopping." How could this be? But, after a while, I got used to it. The pacemaker doesn't hurt, and it helped to prevent me from passing out. So, besides when I must have the battery changed out every 10+ years, having a pacemaker is no big deal compared to other things in my life that I am fighting.

It was during this time, that I was also evaluated by Dr. Blair Grubb in Toledo, Ohio. He was a specialist with patients who had refractory vasovagal syncope. It was there when I learned I had another condition called "Ehlers-Danlos Syndrome." In addition to my fluid balance issues causing the near-syncopal episodes, I also had extremely flexible joints. For instance, I can move my thumb upside down and parallel to my wrist. Note: This isn't normal! Dr. Grubb did all sorts of testing, and then finally told me that "You just weren't put together right. I can't put my finger on it all, but your body just isn't built normal."

This one appointment gave me many things to think about while my Mom and I drove 3 hours back home. The Ehlers-Danlos Syndrome with Hypermobility, was a diagnosis that I would soon forget. So, what if my joints were hypermobile? What difference would that make? Well, changes to my connective tissue would become apparent, as this is associated with this type of syndrome. But, I didn't have issues with that until many years later. Dr. Grubb did agree that working 12-16hr days was something my body couldn't handle. And, he suggested that I get a desk position as a nurse. He also gave me some suggestions as to what else may help to control these dizzy episodes, even after the pacemaker was in place. He tweaked my pacemaker settings, and that finally fixed most of my issues with the near-fainting spells.

Eventually, things started to turn around again. After the pacemaker was placed, I decided that the SICU was not the place I should continue working in due to the incredibly long 12-16 hour shifts. I loved the upbeat pace of that unit, but I saw some very difficult situations, and some extremely sick people. This trauma unit truly saw the sickest of the sick…we got the traumas, life flights, neuro, burns, etc. Anyone that was critically ill was in the SICU. It was an extremely stressful work environment, and I could never manage to get my brain to "turn off." My body did not adjust well to the night shift either, especially when I would get mandated to stay over. So, I began my search for a different nursing position.

I found a job opening at OSU East hospital…a small, rural, community hospital that was still a part of The Ohio State University, but located in a rural part of town. The position was for an RN in Endoscopy. Endoscopy is a department where you take care of inpatients and outpatients who undergo short gastrointestinal procedures. The position was a day-time position, with some on-call responsibilities. I got an interview almost immediately with that department. My ICU experience would come in handy, as these patients undergo conscious sedation, which carries some risks anytime anesthesia is used. I was offered the position, and transferred to that hospital in October of 2003.

I worked with patients who needed procedures done…most of the time our patients had either an EGD or a Colonoscopy. Working with conscious sedation patients required extra knowledge about airways, ventilator support, sedation training, anticipation before someone crashes, BLS/ACLS, etc. This unit was the perfect fit for me, and I felt like I had finally found my niche in nursing.

I love working with GI patients….especially, being able to work with inpatients and outpatients. We see walky-talky, healthy patients, as well as, some extremely sick patients (like the ones I took care of in the ICU). It is a good mix, and never gets boring at all. There is always something to do, something new to learn every day, and the work days go by quickly. We have an amazing staff, which helps tremendously, as that is what has kept me in this field for so long! In fact, I transferred to Grant Medical Center in 2010, with the same GI doctors that I started working with to continue my career in Gastroenterology.

Initially, two gastroenterologists started the GI Lab, Dr. Tasos Manokas and Dr. Adam Tzagournis. These are the two most passionate and caring individuals I have ever met. We have fun with our patients, make them laugh, and do everything possible to make them comfortable during their procedure. I always treat my patients with the dignity and respect that I, myself, would want to be treated as a patient.

Our number one priority is the patient, and making sure they are safe, comfortable, and have a positive experience. Explaining to a patient that a scope will go down their throat, up their bottom, or into their small intestine can be extremely scary to a patient. Somehow, I have been able to wipe away their fears, put the patients at ease, and we have been able to give them the best experience possible during a time when they are the most vulnerable. It takes a special person to do this kind of work every day.

I have never felt like this was truly "work" because we always have a good day, no matter how busy we are. Our team of doctors, nurses, CRNA's, and anesthesiologists always work extremely well together. We do our best to ease the fear that our patients have prior to their procedure. These patients come back years later, and remember our names. Our patients give us extremely positive feedback and outstanding reviews.

In March of 2004, I ended up having some vague GI symptoms myself: heartburn, nausea, cramping, abdominal pain just under my ribs on the right upper side of my abdomen. My GI doctor did a few tests, including a HIDA scan. This scan looks at the function of the gallbladder. The results of this test showed that my gallbladder was beginning to fail. How was this possible at the age of 24? I didn't fit the criteria at all for a gallbladder issue (fat, female, forty---the 3 f's is what we call it). I had an EGD to make sure that I didn't have an ulcer.....the only thing that they saw was a lot of bile at the time, which was irritating my stomach lining.

I ended up having surgery to remove my gallbladder that spring of 2004. I remember waking up in the PACU with extremely, uncontrolled pain in my abdomen. My surgery only lasted 20 minutes…. I asked my surgeon if he just made a cut and ripped my gallbladder out, because that is what it felt like! Why was I in SO much pain? The IV pain medicine was not working. The nurses had given me so much that they thought I would quit breathing. However, my heart rate was over 100 beats/min., and my blood pressure was extremely elevated. I obviously was in pain, and my body was showing other outward signs of it. Due to the extreme pain issue, I ended up being admitted overnight for observation.

The surgeon tried multiple medications to get my pain under control, however, nothing seemed to help. Then, I began having issues with nausea……not just a little bit….a lot! Unfortunately, the doctor didn't know exactly what was wrong, and discharged me with follow-up appointments within a few weeks.

One morning at work, I was working in the recovery room with two other nurses. It was a typical day…. we were trying to get 30 patients done with only 4 bays available for use. I recall starting an IV on a patient to get them prepped for a procedure when something strange happened. An extremely intense pain came on in my stomach. It hurt so much that it took my breath away and doubled me over, and I almost passed out from such severe pain. My co-workers sat me down in a chair, and got me a cool washcloth for my forehead. The pain got even worse and more intense, to the point that I thought I was having a heart attack in my stomach. I attempted to continue to work, thinking it was some irritable bowel symptoms. But, I got another severe pain attack in my stomach, became extremely pale, light-headed, and almost passed out. My manager wheeled me down to the Emergency Room, where nurses hooked me up to a monitor, gave me some pain medicine, and sent me for some tests and x-rays.

Labs came back fine. Abdominal x-rays came back normal. Ct scan came back normal. This just didn't make sense. I truly felt like I was having a heart attack in my stomach. The doctors ended up admitting me, where I ended up spending ~two weeks in the hospital going from test, after test, after test. Nothing was giving them a good explanation as to why I was having so much pain in my stomach that one day, and it was also happening every time after I would eat. My gallbladder was normal, except for some delayed emptying issues.

My GI doctors were stumped. One morning, a medical management team doctor came in after every test was coming back normal, I remember him asking me, "Every test we have performed has come back normal, yet you continue to say that you are having this severe pain intermittently. Do you think that you may be depressed? Did you *really* have that much pain?"

Well, that just about did it. I was SO mad that he inferred that I may be depressed, faking an illness, or that this pain was "all in my head." The excruciating pain that I had that morning at work *was* real! It *was* the most intense pain ever! I truly felt like I was having a heart attack in my stomach. Therefore, I told this ignorant MD that I was NOT depressed, and that they needed to figure out what was wrong with me. Something just wasn't right......they just had not found it yet.

After this run-in with that physician, I immediately called my GI doctor who was working downstairs in the GI lab. I was furious that someone would accuse me of either faking an illness or being depressed. I was crying because I was so extremely upset with what that doctor had just said to me. I was also getting very frustrated because we weren't finding a cause for the severe abdominal pain, along with these other vague symptoms. Dr. Manokas, my GI doctor, convinced me to stay one more day in the hospital because he wanted to have one more test run....an Abdominal Angiogram to look at the major blood vessels around my stomach and intestines.

My mom and I went back and forth as to whether this angiogram was necessary. However, I knew something wasn't right. No one should feel like they are having a heart attack in their stomach, and think that there is absolutely nothing wrong. I knew that something was wrong... they just had not performed the right test yet. So, I agreed to do this last procedure and prayed that something would show up to prove I wasn't crazy or depressed. Then, I asked to speak to the nurse manager on the floor because I wanted that ignorant medical management physician to be discharged from my case. I didn't need him in my room stirring the pot any more than he already had. He was removed from my case, and the angiogram was scheduled for the next morning.

Lying flat on a very cold table, hooked up to lots of monitors, I remember an extremely, caring interventional radiologist talking to me about my symptoms. Then, he explained what they were looking at... the blood vessels in my abdomen. This test would show if any of the arteries were narrowed or deformed in any way, which would explain the symptoms I was having.

After signing the consent form, the nurses pushed some medicine through my IV to help me relax during the procedure. The next thing I remember, I looked over and saw the interventional radiologist talking with my GI doctor. They both were looking at my scans in disbelief. I got the feeling that something just wasn't right. However, I kept drifting in and out of consciousness because of the sedation, so I wasn't awake enough to really pay attention to what all was going on.

Before sending me back to the floor, the interventional radiologist came over and told me what was going on. Indeed, the scan showed an abnormality to explain the extreme pain. I had something very rare called "Median Arcuate Ligament Syndrome." A large, fibrous ligament band was wrapped around my superior mesenteric artery and iliac arteries. This meant that every time I exhaled, this fibrous band was causing very constricted blood flow to my stomach and intestines. In fact, the blood flow was so constricted at times, there was concern that these organs possibly weren't receiving enough blood flow, which would compromise my small intestines.

Finally! We found the answer as to what was causing all of my symptoms. The only problem was this condition is extremely rare. There were only 57 known cases of this condition around the entire world! Fifty-seven cases......that was it!! With my diagnosis, I made #58. Since this condition was so rare, finding a vascular surgeon who was highly experienced in this condition, would be nearly impossible to find.

Once we knew what was causing the pain, the hospital discharged me home because there wasn't anything else they could do there at a small, community hospital. I was going to need surgery. But, in the meantime, they told me to rest, and not do anything that could potentially send me into such a bad flare again. Physical stress could easily place me at risk for another flare, so I had to be very careful in my daily activities to not recreate a stressful, fast-paced situation that would set off another severe stomach attack.

Dr. William Smead, an incredible vascular surgeon, at The Ohio State University, was familiar with my disease. However, he had treated a handful of patients with superior mesenteric artery(SMA) syndrome, where just the SMA artery is compressed. But, he had no experience with someone who had both arteries compressed like what I had. However, the principle as to how to treat it was generally the same. Most likely, I probably wasn't going to be able to find a surgeon who performed this exact surgery in the past because only 57 cases existed in the entire world! Dr. Smead thought there was a chance that only my SMA was involved, but wouldn't know for sure until he had me in the OR and could see for himself as to what exactly this fibrous band was constricting. The only two options during the surgery were:

- Cut the fibrous band to allow the blood to flow properly throughout my stomach and small intestines
- Bypass the area completely using grafts (very complicated)

Luckily, my surgeon was able to cut the large fibrous bands away from the arteries to allow the blood to flow properly. There is always a chance that the fibrous bands could grow back. However, so far, so good (knock on wood)!

The abdominal surgery was a very large surgery. I had an incision that started just below my sternum and went all the way down to the middle of my abdomen. The incision was approximately 10 inches long! I recall that my recovery was quite difficult, as all the muscles around the incision were cut for my surgeon to get visualization of the affected area.

The biggest issue I had during recovery was with eating…or lack thereof. I wasn't very hungry at all after the surgery for multiple weeks. And, I couldn't eat very much without getting nauseated or throwing up. I filled up very quickly and began losing a lot of weight…. weight that I didn't have to lose. I am tall, 5ft7in., and normally weigh around 135 lbs. Despite trying an all liquid diet, I was still unable to keep anything down. I was so nauseated all the time and completely miserable!

Over the course of the next few weeks, I was in and out of the hospital due to dehydration. My GI doctor ended up scoping me a few weeks after surgery. EGD's showed a ton of inflammation in my stomach, along with lots and lots of bile(500ml+). This meant that food and fluids were not moving very well out of my system, causing the severe nausea, vomiting, and feeling of fullness.

Initially, the doctors thought that the delayed emptying of my stomach was due to just having such a large abdominal surgery, and my bowels just needed to "wake up." After a month of losing weight, along with constant nausea, vomiting, abdominal pain, and the feeling of fullness despite eating almost nothing, Dr. Manokas realized that I was dealing with something much more serious than just post-op issues. More than likely, I was dealing with gastroparesis!

The vagus nerve is a major nerve that enables the stomach to contract, which helps to propel food through the stomach and into the small intestine. Obviously, the vagus nerve was injured in some way during the surgery to ligate the ligament/fibrous band that was wrapped around several main arteries. This meant that the one nerve that controls the emptying and contracting of my stomach was not working properly, if at all. To confirm this diagnosis, my doctor ordered a gastric emptying study.

The gastric emptying study required me to drink an 8oz. glass of liquid oatmeal. I recall it was so difficult to even get that down due to the severe nausea and full feeling. They gave me only ~10 minutes to drink it, and then they would begin the scan. Trying to get that liquid oatmeal (containing the radiopaque dye) down was awful, but I knew I needed to do my best to figure out what was going on. I was finally able to get all the liquid oatmeal down, and then I had to lie flat on a hard mattress for about an hour while a machine hovered over my abdomen and scanned my stomach.

Once the gastric emptying study was complete, it confirmed Dr. Manokas' suspicion that I had gastroparesis. My gastric emptying study showed that my stomach emptying time was 5x slower than normal for digesting liquids. If it was that slow emptying just liquids, I couldn't imagine how long it was taking for solid food to empty out of my stomach! Finally, an answer as to what was causing all of these issues post-surgery. There was a chance that the gastroparesis could go into remission. However, I was told that if that was going to happen, it most likely would happen within the first year of being diagnosed with gastroparesis.

As a nurse in the gastroenterology department, I discussed this diagnosis so many times with newly diagnosed gastroparesis patients, but little did I ever think that I would become a GI patient myself. At the age of 24, I was experiencing all the awful symptoms that gastroparesis patients would report. Extreme nausea was the most bothersome symptom for me. I always said that if I could just throw-up, I'd feel so much better. I would vomit sometimes, but most of the time, I had severe, persistent nausea that didn't respond to any medical treatment.

My doctor tried just about every medication possible to help with symptoms of severe nausea, vomiting, weight loss, and acid reflux…. Reglan, Domperidone, Erythromycin, Zithromax, Phenergan, Zofran, Compazine, Marinol, Prevacid, Nexium, Zantac, Zegarid, etc. The list goes on and on. I ended up having "refractory gastroparesis" meaning my condition was not able to be treated with the standard medication regimen alone.

I spent many days, nights, and holidays in the hospital due to the gastroparesis. I would have "flare-ups" when I was sick with a virus or even a common cold. The tiniest of things would set it off even worse. During flare-ups, I was restricted to an all liquid diet for 3 or more days to give my stomach a rest, and then we would slowly reintroduce a gastroparesis diet again. Sometimes this would work…. other times, I would end up in the ER receiving IV fluids.

The medications that truly worked best for me were Zithromax, Domperidone, Zofran, and Phenergan. Zithromax suspension of 200mg twice a day, helped with the contractions of my stomach. Even though it was an antibiotic, a side effect of it was stomach cramps. So, many GI doctors were using it to treat gastroparesis. I was able to be on this medicine for over two years without any side effects, and it did help move things through my GI tract better.

Domperidone is a medication that I also tried initially. It is only available in Canada, though. My doctor would write a script for it, fax it to the pharmacy in Canada, and then it would have to pass border patrol to arrive here in the United States. There were several times that my medication was confiscated at the border, which was so frustrating when I needed the medication. Despite letters and pleas to the border patrol, we ended up deciding this was not the best situation, and we needed to figure out another way to get this medication easier without the hassle of border patrol agents. My GI doctor had learned that domperidone could be made here in the United States, by getting it from a compounding pharmacy.

Most states have a compounding pharmacy. They can compound any medication out there with a prescription from the doctor. This turned out to be the better way to go. However, it was very expensive doing it this way. Eventually, my body would get used to each pro-motility drug and I would get to the maximum doses on each medication.

This meant that we had to switch things up and try another motility drug and other alternative treatments.

One of the very first procedures I had was an EGD with Botox. It is an endoscopic procedure done to look at the esophagus, stomach, and first portion of the small bowel. During the scope, my doctor injected Botox, a muscle paralytic, into the pylorus muscle to keep the end of my stomach open. This allowed liquids and food to drain much easier, which ultimately helped my symptoms of gastroparesis go away. I would get a good 10-12 weeks of relief out of this, and then I would have to return for the same procedure again. I think I had around 40 EGD's total in a 10-year time period!

At one point, my insurance company started denying treatment with the Botox. They said that Botox was not FDA approved for gastroparesis, therefore, they couldn't continue to let me have this procedure. I was so devastated! These procedures were the only thing keeping me out of the hospital all the time! We tried everything possible…wrote letters of medical necessity, spoke to the doctor who made this decision, and did a peer to peer review, etc. He wouldn't budge on his ruling, and refused to allow the EGD with Botox procedures to continue. What would we do now?

My gastroenterologist had to think about this a little, as did I. I was brainstorming other options. I thought about other similar procedures we did in endoscopy. When a patient would come in with a stricture(narrowing) in their esophagus or in their colon, we would use a specific balloon that fits through the scope to "open up" the stricture. Why couldn't we do this for the stomach?

I presented the idea to Dr. Manokas, and he agreed that it was something we could try. Companies did make specific pyloric balloons, so there was a balloon out there specifically for this. All we needed to do was make sure we ordered the correct size balloon to be able to open that area at the end of my stomach as much as possible.

I didn't have a stricture, necessarily. However, it made sense that this was something we could try. The next time I needed my stomach to be dilated, we tried this pyloric balloon and it worked!!!! I was SO happy that we figured out something else to use besides the Botox. I would also have this done over the course of several years. They wouldn't usually last as long. Most of the time I would only get 8-10 weeks of relief before symptoms returned and I had to be redilated. But, overall, it was a solution to a big problem.

In December of 2005, I had multiple bad flare-ups of my gastroparesis. Nothing was working, and I had lost a ton of weight over a few months. I was down to almost 100lbs. My doctor had to place a temporary NJ tube for tube feedings. I recall the very first NJ tube placement…. Dr. Manokas and Dr. Adam Tzagournis were both at my bedside. One was holding this long; thin tube and the other was there for moral support. They told me I needed the NJ tube to get some nutrition and gain some weight back.

I'm not going to lie, the NJ tube was complete torture! Putting that down my nose was the worst thing ever! Dr. Tzagournis was holding my hands down, while Dr. Manokas put the tube down my nose. One side didn't open up enough, so he had to put it down the other nostril. I remember tears streaming down my face, screaming in pain, and just being angry and frustrated overall.

"Swallow!" I'd hear them say. I tried to swallow, but I felt like I was gagging and choking on the tube. Tears continued to stream down my face from fear and frustration. What had my life come to?

Finally, after multiple attempts, the doctors were able to get the NJ tube placed, and we could start feedings once x-ray cleared it. The NJ tube only bought me some time…it would last a few days to a week before I would have to have a more permanent solution to help during these periods of gastroparesis flare ups.

December 23, 2005…two days before Christmas, I ended up having to have a j-tube surgically placed. I had lost so much weight, that the NJ tube for a week wasn't enough time to gain enough weight back. So, the solution was to surgically place a j-tube. The surgery itself wasn't too bad. It did take some time for my small intestine to cooperate with the tube feedings. I was placed on 24-hour tube feedings for 3 months at that point.

Initially, the rate of the feeds started out at 10ml/hr. They had to slowly increase the rate because my intestines fought the increase every time. I would get extremely bloated, and my intestines wanted to twist around where the tube was placed. Eventually, after two weeks of slowly titrating the rate up, I was at my goal rate of 65ml/hr. I spent Christmas and New Year's in the hospital that year. It was a very rough time. But, the j-tube was the answer at that time to help keep me out of the hospital.

Finally, after about three weeks, I was able to go home. I was hooked up to tube feedings 24 hours a day for three months. I slowly began to eat, in addition to the tube feeds. We weaned the feeds down to nocturnal only at that point. Once I was able to gain enough weight back, and prove that I could maintain my nutrition during the day, we were able to go to tube feedings as needed only depending on how my day was going.

It was very difficult initially with the j-tube. I was super self-conscious of this tube hanging out of my belly. But, at the same time, I was thankful too. I no longer needed to worry about getting enough nutrition in, if I was having a rough day. If my gastroparesis acted up and I couldn't eat much during the day, I was able to do bolus feeds or nocturnal feeds as needed. My GI doctor was very flexible once I got to this point. As a nurse, I knew how to properly take care of the j-tube, and how to count calories to determine what rate I needed to run the tube feedings at during the night.

Eventually, the gastroparesis symptoms slowly got better with time. In November of 2008, I was able to have the j-tube removed. I developed a fistula though, which is a tract that formed from my intestine to my skin. Because of the fistula tract, that hole wouldn't close on its own. I had to have it surgically closed, and then the incision site healed completely on its own.

Once the j-tube was removed, I felt like a new person. I felt like I got my life back. I could swim in the ocean, eat food again, and wear clothes without being self-conscious about how I looked now that the tube was gone. I still had gastroparesis. However, the symptoms were not nearly as severe as they were when the j-tube was in place.

Nearly 3 years passed of being "tube free" when I developed a severe case of gastroparesis after a bad viral infection. I ended up hospitalized for weeks again. My GI doctor did an EGD with balloon dilatation of the pylorus. However, it didn't work that time. They felt that I had SO many procedures, that the pylorus was scarred down now, which is why the EGD with dilatation did not work anymore. This meant that I had to have an NJ tube placed again. We were hoping that I could do temporary tube feedings again, until my stomach decided to wake up. However, after two weeks of having the NJ tube, I ended up with ulcers running down the back of my throat. It was obvious that I needed to be admitted to the hospital for fluid resuscitation, and a new plan of action needed to be made.

Ultimately, it was decided that surgery was necessary at that point. In October of 2010, Dr. Manilchuk was the surgeon on my case. He came into my room and we talked extensively about what the plan was. His concern, as well as mine and the GI doctors as well, was that with a pyloroplasty, I could end up with dumping syndrome or severe bile reflux. This meant that my situation could end up even worse than what it already was. But, there was a chance that it could make things better. I was putting my faith in the doctors, and the good lord above, that things would finally go in my favor. Dr. Manilchuk took three days to think about how he wanted to proceed with my surgery, and carefully thought out each step.

It was ultimately decided that I would have a pyloroplasty with small bowel resection with a roux-n-y anastomosis for j-tube placement; along with lysis of adhesions. This was a huge surgery, that would change my life forever. Once you make a change and widen the pylorus, there is nothing you can do to change it back. Either things would get better, or they would get much, much worse. It was a "crap shoot" for sure. My parents and I were very nervous about this decision. However, things were already going downhill as it was, and I couldn't keep living this way. A j-tube alone would not solve my issues permanently. So, I signed the consent form and off to surgery I went.

When I woke up from surgery, I remember that I was extremely sore. I had multiple incisions and tubes everywhere. I had an incision down the mid-line of my abdomen, as well as, another incision for a fresh new j-tube site. The j-tube was placed because of the viral illness…my stomach wasn't waking up and I needed additional nutritional support at the time. I had an NG tube coming out of my nose to keep stomach contents empty until my bowels woke up from the anesthesia. Initially, this tube drained liters of bile every day…. this was NOT a good sign at all. The complication of severe bile reflux was in the back of my mind as I laid in bed and watched the bile get sucked out of my stomach. Thick, dark green bile was being sucked up and out of my stomach via the NG tube, and then went into the suction canister that was above my bed. The doctors were very concerned about how much bile was being suctioned out every day, as well as how much was draining from my j-tube. Was this a mistake? Was this surgery a huge failure?

As the days went on, I started to feel better. I was still extremely sore and weak from such a large abdominal surgery, but I was hungry. My bowels woke up, the bile drainage began to decrease significantly, and the NG tube was then able to be removed. Tube feedings were started to get my nutrition and protein built back up to heal from the surgery. Then, I could have full liquids to drink. Once I proved that I could drink liquids without getting sick, I was progressed to a gastroparesis diet.

One day I realized that I had absolutely no nausea....... I couldn't believe it! I had lived the past 10+ years with severe nausea every day. Now, I was having no issues at all.... not even one hint of nausea! It appeared that the surgery was not a failure. It was a HUGE success!!!!! I would be that 10% that didn't end up with dumping syndrome or severe bile reflux. I was able to eat normally again. And, I was able to get off all anti-nausea and pro-motility drugs! I couldn't have been happier!

At my follow-up appointment with my surgeon, we discussed exactly what he did during my surgery. One of the things he mentioned was that in addition to what we had talked about prior to surgery, he said that he decided to cut the ligament of Trietz. This was extremely important, and appeared to be a brilliant decision. This allowed my bowels to drop down, which obviously prevented any issues with nausea, bile reflux, etc. I gave Dr. Manilchuk the biggest hug! He gave me my miracle that I had been waiting over 10 years for! Tears streamed down my face once I realized that my nightmare with gastroparesis was ending! I did so well after this surgery, that the j-tube wasn't even needed. It was removed in March of 2011.

Over six years later, I am still nausea-free! It has been such a blessing! I had struggled to survive with severe gastroparesis issues for well over 10 years. Currently, I have flare-ups here and there. I am dealing with bile-reflux issues, and strictures in my esophagus. But, I do not have nausea on a constant basis. Domperidone is the medication that I take currently.

I can eat more than just a gastroparesis diet. I have to follow a gluten-free diet now, because over the last couple of years, it was discovered that I also have a gluten allergy, also known as Celiac disease. This means that I must avoid any foods that contain gluten.

Gluten is found in wheat, rye, barley, and oats. It is in a ton of processed food, and is in practically anything that tastes good! Learning to eat a gluten-free diet was a challenge, but it has gotten easier as time has gone on. I have learned through several doctors, that Celiac disease is actually becoming more and more common to have in conjunction with gastroparesis.

Hopefully, my life story helps to lift your spirits and gives you hope. There is a chance that things *will* get better for you! A life with gastroparesis is very difficult, no doubt. But, there are many medications and treatments out there that help control the severe symptoms of gastroparesis. Everyone reacts to things differently. What may work well for one person, may not help another, and vice versa. But, miracles do happen…. I am living proof of that!

While I am mainly cured from gastroparesis, I have continued to fight several other debilitating conditions, including MCAS and RSD/CRPS. RSD/CRPS stands for "Reflex Sympathetic Dystrophy" or is also known as "Chronic Regional Pain Syndrome." This is an extremely painful, debilitating, autoimmune disease that causes lots of damage to the sympathetic nervous system and results in extremely severe burning pain, in addition to a lot of other symptoms. It is the most painful disorder out there…and rates even higher than a person with an amputation. The only way I can describe how RSD/CRPS feels like is: It feels like my left foot and ankle have been doused with lighter fluid and set on fire, and I'm not able to put the fire out.

Unfortunately, I got this most painful disease because of trauma suffered from a broken foot/ankle that happened when I was working as a nurse in the endoscopy department. On May 30, 2008, I was injured at work on a day that I was supposed to be off. However, I worked for a co-worker, so he could take his family on a camping trip. It was *that* day that I was injured.

Several nurses and I were bringing equipment back from a procedure in a train-like fashion, when the nurse in front of me stopped very quickly and caused a chain reaction. I got caught in the middle, and the cart that was being pushed behind me caught the back of my left foot/ankle and turned it upside down. I had four avulsion (twisted bone) fractures, as well as a Lisfranc injury. In addition to the four fractures in my foot and ankle, I also tore all the ligaments across the top of my foot. Since this happened at work, all treatments had to get approved through workers compensation. This meant many, many, many delays. By the time I was able to get approved to see an orthopedic doctor, I had already gone into RSD/CRPS. There was nothing the orthopedic doctor could do. Surgery would be extremely risky. RSD/CRPS causes significantly decreased blood flow to the injury site. If I had surgery to correct the ligament damage, I would have been at very high risk of losing my foot due to decreased circulation.

With RSD/CRPS, the body senses the trauma, but continues to sense it way beyond a normal healing time. This results in a non-stop cycle of extremely severe pain, inflammation, bony changes, osteoporosis, skin changes, temperature changes, and nail changes in the affected extremity. It is known to spread to other extremities, and can go full body and invade the organs as well. Many patients with this disease end up disabled and in a wheelchair. RSD/CRPS is extremely rare. It is the most severe, debilitating disease out there. As of right now, there is no cure for RSD/CRPS. While I am not dealing with the severe gastroparesis any more, I am fighting for my life every single day due to the RSD/CRPS. Unfortunately, I have traded one severely debilitating disease for another!

In February of 2015, I was given the opportunity of a lifetime to see the top specialist in this field, Dr. Pradeep Chopra in Pawtucket, RI. He treated my RSD/CRPS, but also diagnosed MCAS and Ehlers-Danlos Syndrome Type III. It was at this appointment, that my life changed forever.

Dr. Chopra put me on the right path for treating the RSD/CRPS. I actually into remission, which is really unheard of, within 3 months of seeing Dr.Chopra. I needed to take additional supplements like Vitamin C and Magnesium. He also switched some medications around, and placed me on a medication called LDN. It helps to control my immune system, which plays a huge role in all of my conditions. I continued daily exercise and walking. And, I followed the MCAS protocol. In May of 2015, I WAS in true remission from RSD/CRPS. I no longer had any pain, color changes, temperature changes, or anything else associated with this condition.

It was at this appointment that I learned that everything I had been through my entire life was tied together by one condition, Ehlers-Danlos Syndrome. Dr. Chopra put the puzzle pieces together. Autonomic dysfunction, Median Arcuate Ligament Dysfunction, Gastroparesis, Celiac Disease, RSD/CRPS, MCAS, and Ehlers-Danlos Syndrome were ALL tied together. This was the answer that I needed.

In September of 2015, I was able to return to work as an RN, CGRN in the GI department at Grant Medical Center. I continue to work here full-time to this day. I have been recognized as a senior GI specialist in my department, and continue to help to mentor many co-workers and patients on different conditions. Unfortunately, in October of 2017, I fell out of remission with my RSD/CRPS after having a stent placed in my left common iliac vein for May-Thurner Syndrome. Despite this set-back, I REFUSE to give up HOPE. Remission IS possible again!

I just hope and pray that one day everything will be ok. My health history is extremely complex for someone so young. However, my outlook and attitude remains the same. Although there is not a cure out there for RSD/CRPS, as well as gastroparesis, I remain hopeful. Researchers are constantly working to find cures for these diseases every day. They are getting closer and closer to finding a cure. This truly gives me hope.

If you have HOPE, anything is possible! Miracles happen each and every day. You never know when YOU will be the one to finally catch a break and go into remission from whatever ails you. Living with a chronic disease is extremely tough physically, mentally, and emotionally. It is so very important to maintain a good support system, keep a positive attitude, and remain hopeful as hard as it may be at times. Where there is hope…. anything is possible! Miracles happen every day. You never know….one day *You* may be the next recipient of a miracle!!

13

Coping Methods:

Pet Therapy, Guided Imagery, and Music Therapy

Everyone needs an "outlet" when dealing with a chronic illness. Living with a chronic illness, like gastroparesis, can completely zap all of your energy from you. You may become more isolated, frustrated, and irritable due to the constant symptoms of chronic nausea, vomiting, fatigue, and lack of sleep. You might find yourself sleeping more than you used to prior to getting gastroparesis. These feelings are all normal.

However, these feelings can also lead people down a spiraling path where they feel completely hopeless and isolate themselves. This in turn usually leads to depression. If left untreated, depression can lead to suicide. I must be very honest and mention this because this is reality. Living with a chronic illness is not easy, and is extremely tough physically, mentally, and emotionally. Therefore, it is extremely important that you have a good support system and utilize different coping methods to help deal with these feelings daily. An evaluation by a psychologist may be necessary at some point to help you express your feelings, and learn which is the best way to cope with these issues.

Over the years, I have realized just how important it is to take some time out of the day just for *you*. Even if that means just taking a short walk, going to a yoga class, reading a good book, sitting outside at a park, or watching a good movie. These things are therapeutic and highly recommended when you are dealing with a serious chronic illness on a daily basis. But, I also recommend that you learn some different coping methods as well. Try to focus your mind on something else other than your gastroparesis symptoms. Consider utilizing some coping skills such as: pet therapy, guided imagery, or music therapy.

Pet Therapy

Pet therapy can play a very important role in the life of anyone who is dealing with a chronic condition daily. Overall, taking care of a pet or visiting with a pet can help you mentally and emotionally. You build a very special bond between the two of you….a bond that is unique just for *You*.

Pet therapy is gaining attention in the healthcare field and beyond. If you are admitted to a hospital, usually the hospital has an animal-assisted activity for providing comfort to their patients. Usually, your nurse or doctor should mention this program to you and ask if you want to participate. If you agree to participate, an assistance dog and its owner will visit you in your hospital room. They typically stay 10-15 minutes, and allow you to pet the dog and interact with the animal, as well as, its owner too.

Afterwards, you probably will find yourself smiling and feeling a little less tired. And, hopefully, feel a little bit more optimistic too. It gives you something to talk about to your family and friends. And, the dog will come back and visit you throughout your stay in the hospital.

I remember when I was admitted to the hospital for a few weeks over the holidays due to a severe gastroparesis flare-up. My j-tube was inserted during that time, and we had to slowly increase the tube feedings. During my stay, I was able to have a pet therapy dog come and visit me every couple of days. The dog looked like a Benjie dog, and her name was Rosie. Rosie was as sweet as she could be and extremely gentle. She was very well mannered, and let me pet her as she laid right next to me in the bed. The dog's owner was an older woman, who was very sociable as well. The overall experience was very positive and something I looked forward to! It lifted my spirits every day that I was in the hospital!!

Multiple studies have shown that pet therapy can significantly reduce pain, anxiety, depression, and fatigue in patients who are dealing with a wide range of health problems. Obviously, the biggest concern is safety and sanitation. However, most hospitals and facilities have very strict rules to ensure that the animals are all vaccinated and well trained.

Many hospitals have over a dozen certified pet therapy dogs that are part of its pet therapy program. These dogs make regular visits to different departments, and can even make special visits on request. One example that the Mayo Clinic reported is about one dog and his trainer that worked with a young 5-year-old girl who was recovering from surgery on her spine. The pet therapy dog helped her relearn how to walk! For each step that she took forward, the therapy dog would take a step backwards. (18). Just thinking about this puts a smile on my face!

It is remarkable what these dogs are trained to do. Pet therapy is extremely beneficial to both the patient and the dog. So, the next time you must be in the hospital, please know that these pet therapy programs do exist, and they can definitely help to improve your mood and lift your spirits.

Pet therapy can also include having a pet of your own to care for, whether it is a dog or a cat. An animal that you are responsible for…that depends on you to feed it, take it outside, go for walks, and care for it on a daily basis can have the same effects that a therapy dog does to patients in the hospital. Overall, having something else to focus your attention on, helps your mental outlook. And, it usually takes your mind away from constantly thinking about your nagging and uncomfortable gastroparesis symptoms. A walk with your dog can do wonders for someone with a chronic illness!

I know I couldn't have made it through everything I've been through without my golden retriever. Bogey had been through everything with me, and had always been there through thick and thin. He is what kept me going, when my health took a turn for the worse. I swear that dog was SO smart, and knew exactly what I was saying when I talked to him. He tried to talk back, by using his vocal cords to "talk" in his own sweet way. Our bond grew tremendously over the past 12 years. Bogey kept me going during some extremely difficult moments in my life. I am forever grateful for this extremely beautiful and loyal companion who "chose" me!

Bogey and I usually took two daily walks a day…this was our "special" time together to walk, relax, let go of our problems, and enjoy the simple things in life. I had to laugh though, because Bogey had about four different walking paths to take, and he decided which way we would go each and every time! Everywhere we walked, each person commented on how beautiful Bogey was, and how friendly he was. Bogey was well-known in my community…. who wouldn't love that cute face with the most beautiful dark brown eyes?!

When Bogey was almost 14 years old, I had to be extremely careful with him in the hot weather, as well as the cold weather too. His body was much more fragile than when he was younger….and it took him longer to recover from a walk But, despite some hip issues, and some cancerous lumps all over his body, this dog continued to push on. We took two walks a day, and I enjoyed each and every minute of it. I loved watching him enjoy just the simple things in life…. the smells of freshly cut grass, beautiful flowers, enjoying the warm sunshine, and constantly sniffing the grass and the air when those gentle breezes come and go..

Bogey was that extremely special bond for me! Who knew that this $35 dog at the pound would turn out to be seriously the best dog ever?!? Below, is a precious picture of my dog, Bogey! He was ~14 years old in this picture. Those eyes tell SO much….such a sweet soul with a heart of gold!!!!

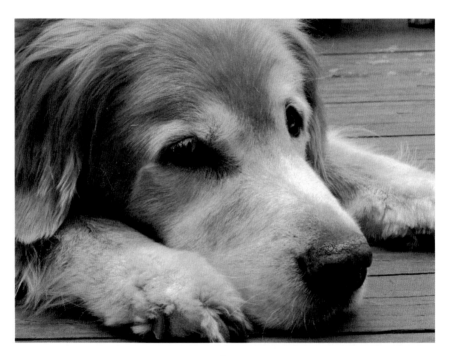

My dearest Bogey…You've been my rock, my inspiration, my protector, my best buddy, and the most loyal, trusting companion anyone could ask for. I have been truly blessed to have you in my life for the past 12+ years. I am SO lucky that you chose *me* to be your Mom!!!!! We've been through an awful lot together! Thank You for *always* standing by my side, and helping get me through some very tough times!!!

Without Bogey, I would not be the person I am today. He taught me patience, love, loyalty, strength, determination, and unconditional love. I am so glad that I took that chance many years ago, and gave him the ability to show me just how strong, gentle, and loving a male dog can be!

Bogey passed away shortly after I finished writing the majority of this book. September 29, 2014 is a day I will never forget. It is the day I laid my boy to rest and set him free. No more pain, no more suffering. As hard as that day was, I know it was the right decision. Bogey completed his mission here on earth. He did SO much more than what anyone could ask of a dog. I was truly blessed to have him in my life! I love you to the moon and back, Bogey!!!! I look forward to meeting up with you again at "The Rainbow Bridge." Until then, I promise to carry on your legacy and live life to the fullest!

~`~`~`~`~`~`~`

Guided Imagery

Another coping mechanism patients with chronic illnesses find helpful is using guided imagery. "Guided imagery is a form of meditation that draws upon the power of guided imagery to help you enter into a state of deep relaxation and mental stillness. It is one of the simplest and most powerful ways to eliminate stress, and to experience total inner peace." (19)

Guided imagery is a wonderful and easy way to relax and focus your mind on something pleasant. Anyone can experience a state of relaxation and deep meditation using guided imagery. You can do this at any time and any place. All you have to do is find a comfortable place to sit, put on some headphones, and play the guided imagery CD. This will allow yourself to be guided into a state of deep relaxation and meditation while listening to soothing music and a narrator.

As you listen to the guided imagery CD, you will be asked to visualize several different scenes that have a calming effect on your mind, body, and entire nervous system. During the meditation, your muscles will relax, your breathing will be easy, your blood pressure and heart rate will normalize, your immune system function will improve, and your emotions will settle down. By imagining positive, soothing experiences, your entire body becomes relaxed and releases natural chemicals that make you feel more optimistic. Overall, most patients find guided imagery to be extremely beneficial after the session is completed. (19).

There are many guided imagery CD's available, as well as, some free ones if you just google "guided imagery" on your phone apps. The nice thing about guided imagery is that it is something you can do in a relatively short amount of time (~20 minutes), and you can do it several times a day, as needed.

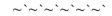

Music Therapy

Lastly, another coping mechanism that can be tried to take your mind off of being sick all of the time, is through the use of music therapy. Music therapy works a lot like guided imagery, except you are listening to music instead. Music therapy can include creating, singing, moving to, and/or listening to music.

Music is a form of sensory stimulation, which creates certain responses in the body such as: improved breathing rate, lowered blood pressure, improved heart function, reduced heart rate, reduced pain levels, and relaxed muscle tension. (20).

Music takes the person away from all the problems that currently ails them, and allows them to drift into another world of calm and peacefulness. There are many ways in which this can be done. However, if you are at home, all you need to do is find a comfortable spot to lie down, put on some headphones, and turn on your favorite, relaxing music. After allowing yourself to drift off into another place for about 20 minutes, you should notice your body is in a much more relaxed state than when you began the music therapy (20).

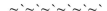

Living with a severe chronic medical condition is extremely taxing on the mind, body, and spirit. It is so important that you find yourself an "outlet." A place and an activity that takes your mind away from constantly thinking about being sick is so extremely important in how you should live day to day. Whether you decide to take a walk, go to a yoga class, swim in the pool, watch a movie, or read a good book.... just have fun and let your mind and body just rest and relax.

Keep in mind that there may be some extremely difficult times in your life too when you may need to add some additional coping methods into your day such as pet therapy, guided imagery, and/or music therapy. These activities are excellent ways to help relax your mind and body, as well as, lift your spirits. This is incredibly important when dealing with a chronic illness day in and day out.

Lastly, the most important thing to do is: Never. Ever. Give. Up. HOPE! With hope, anything is possible! Where there is hope…there are possibilities. Where there are possibilities…there are miracles! Miracles happen each and every day! Keep the faith…. a cure for gastroparesis and other chronic conditions _will_ be found!!!!!!

Additional Resources

Gastroparesis Resources:

www.mayoclinic.org/diseases-conditions/gastroparesis/resources
www.aboutgastroparesis.org/living-with-gastroparesis/resources
www.gastroparesisandme.com
www.medhelp.org/tags/show/3163/gastroparesis
www.emilysstomach.com/2012/12/gastroparesis-resources-online
gpresourcehub.weebly.com
www.aboutgastroparesis.org
www.helpgastroparesis.org/#!
www.aboutgastroparesis.org/treatments/complimentary
gi.org/guideline/management-of-gastroparesis
digestive.niddk.nih.gov/ddiseases/pubs/gastroparesis

Gastroparesis Diet:

gicare.com
www.digestivediseaseny.com/nutrition/gastroparesis
   uvahealth.com/.../image-and-docs/gastroparesis-diet.pdf
www.livestrong>...>DigestiveConditions>Gastroparesis
www.mayoclinic/org/diseases-conditions/gastroparesis/basics/
www.arizonadigestivehealth.com/gastroparesis-diet
www.motilitysociety.org/patient/pdf/Gastroparesis%20AMS%20Dietary

Sample Meals for Gastroparesis:

www.aboutgastroparesis.org/treatments/diet/sample-meal-plans
www.livestrong>DigestiveConditions>Gastroparesis
www.nutrition411.com>PatientEducationMaterials
www.digestivediseaseny.com/nutrition/gastroparesis
www.motilitysociety.org/patient/pdf/Gastroparesis%20AMS%20Dietary
   answers.yahoo.com/question?qd=20120107071708AaeBn1o
www.aboutgastroparesis.org/treatments/diet/recommendations
www.recipes-pro.com/lp1/index.php?k=gastroparesis%20recipes

Conclusion

As this book ends, it is my hope that I have provided you with some helpful information on how to deal with gastroparesis on a daily basis. When I was diagnosed with gastroparesis almost 15 years ago, there was very little information available on this disease. However, I have become quite educated on GI diseases during my career as a certified gastroenterology registered nurse. It is incredible that I can talk with my patients prior to their procedure to let them know exactly what they can expect to hear or feel before, during, and after the procedure. This knowledge as a registered nurse, as well as, a gastroparesis patient, helps to put many patients at ease.

As a gastroparesis patient myself, I know the reality and true struggles that you are going through. Living with gastroparesis 24/7 truly takes everything out of you some days, and makes it difficult to move forward. I hope that my story is an inspiration to you, as well as others, and gives you hope that a cure is on the horizon!

Never..Ever..Give..Up..HOPE!! Remission IS Possible! Anything is possible with HOPE!!!

About the Author

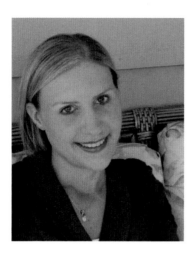

Kathryn M. Rogers is 38 years old and lives in Columbus, Ohio. She graduated from Miami University in Oxford, Ohio in December of 2001 with a Bachelor's of Science in Nursing degree. After college, Katie moved back home to be closer to her family, and begin her life on her own. Katie is a mom to a 3-year-old golden retriever named Riley. She has two brothers and two nephews who also live in Columbus, OH. Katie's parents, her biggest supporters, live nearby in Columbus, Ohio.

Katie began her nursing career as a Registered Nurse at The Ohio State University in the Surgical Intensive Care Unit in March of 2002. After obtaining two years of experience in this intensive setting, Katie chose to change positions and obtained a new position as a gastroenterology nurse. This is when she fell in love with a specific niche in nursing, and continues to work as a certified gastroenterology registered nurse for nearly 13+ years. In 2010, Katie took an extremely difficult gastroenterology certification exam to become certified as a CGRN. She passed the exam, and became the first nurse in her unit to be certified in gastroenterology.

Despite many health issues along the way, Katie continues to move forward and push through each and every day. There were some extremely scary and difficult moments over the past 15 years. Fighting gastroparesis for so many years, while trying to continue working at the same time, was extremely difficult at times…especially when dealing with the surgeries and feeding tubes. Anger and frustration was there, however, Katie did not let it stop her. In 2010, Katie had the surgery that cured her gastroparesis forever. However, just as we thought that the biggest battle had been fought and won, Katie was struck with another extremely rare condition called RSD/CRPS.

Reflex Sympathetic Dystrophy/Chronic Regional Pain Syndrome is by far the most painful condition ever. It causes extreme burning/scalding pain, swelling, sensitivity to touch, bony changes, osteopenia/osteoporosis, skin becomes red/purple(mottled) and cold to the touch; blood vessels are constantly constricting, which decreases blood flow to that extremity. This condition is progressive, degenerative, and extremely debilitating. It can spread beyond the initial injury, and affect everything, including internal organ damage. There currently is no cure for RSD/CRPS.

So, while gastroparesis has been mostly cured, a battle is still being fought…. stronger than ever. Katie continues to fight through each day, despite excruciating scalding, burning pain at times.

God has a plan for everyone. Some experience more issues than others, for unknown reasons. These challenges/illnesses make us stronger as a person. People with chronic illness will have bumps in the road here and there, and hit some road blocks as well. However, no matter what your battle is, try to stay positive and remember that anything is possible with HOPE! Never ever give up hope! Miracles do happen each and every day…Cures *WILL* be found!

BIBLIOGRAPHY

1. Gastroparesis and Diabetes, NIDDK
   https://www.niddk.nih.gov/health-information/health-topics/digestive-diseases/gastroparesis/Pages/facts.aspx

2. Understanding Gastroparesis and Dyspepsia
   https://www.digestivedistress.com

3. URL: https://www.digestivedistress.com

4. Temple Digestive Disease Center
   https://digestive.templehealth.org/

5. World J Gastroenterology 2009 January 7; 15(1): 25-37. World Journal of Gastroenterology ISSN 1007-9327

6. Waseem S, Moshiree B, Draganov PV. Gastroparesis: Current diagnostic challenges and management considerations. *World J Gastroenterology* 2009; 15(1): 25-37.

7. Gastroparesis Food Guide
   https://www.wexnermedicalcenter.edu

8. Total Parenteral Nutrition
   https://www.vh.org/adult/provider/surgery/totalparenteralnutrition

9. Al-Jurf, Adel S. and Karen Dillon "Indications for Total Parenteral Nutrition(TPN)." University of Iowa Virtual Hospital. March 2003 (cited 16 February 2005).

10. Surgical Options for Gastroparesis
    https://www.wjnet.com

11. URL: https://www.medtronic.com/patients/gastroparesis/device/index.htm

12. Medtronic Enterra Therapy
    https://www.medtronic.inc/enterratherapy

13. Abell T, McCallum R, Hocking M, et al. Gastric electrical stimulation for medically refractory gastroparesis. *Gastroenterology.* August 2003; 125(2): 421-428.

14. URL: https://www.gisurgical.com/minimally-invasive-surgery/laproscopic-pyloroplasty

15. Dumping Syndrome
    https://www.webmd.com/digestive-disorders/dumping-syndrome-causes-foods-treatments?page=2

16. MCAS
    URL: https://en.wikipedia.org/wiki/Mast_cell_activation_syndrome

17. Celiac Disease
    URL://ww.mayoclinic.org/diseases-conditions/celiac-disease/symptoms-causes

18. Gastroparesis Resources-Diseases and Conditions-Mayo Clinic
    URL: http://www.mayoclinic.org/diseases-conditions/gastroparesis/basics/definition/con-20023971

19. Guided Imagery
    URL: https:// www.The-Guided-Imagery-Site.com

20. American Music Therapy Association
    URL: https://www.musictherapy.org/